ESSENTIAL ANAESTHESIA

Essential Anaesthesia

F. R. Ellis PhD, MB, ChB, FFARCS

I. T. Campbell MD, FFARCS

University Departments of Anaesthesia,
Leeds and Liverpool

BLACKWELL SCIENTIFIC PUBLICATIONS

OXFORD LONDON EDINBURGH

BOSTON PALO ALTO MELBOURNE

©1986 by
Blackwell Scientific Publications
Editorial offices:
Osney Mead, Oxford, OX2 0EL
8 John Street, London WC1N 2ES
23 Ainslie Place, Edinburgh EH3 6AJ
52 Beacon Street, Boston
  Massachusetts 02108, USA
667 Lytton Avenue, Palo Alto
  California 94301, USA
107 Barry Street, Carlton
  Victoria 3053, Australia

First published 1986

Set by Katerprint Typesetting
Services, Oxford, England.
Printed in Great Britain by
Billing and Sons Ltd,
Worcester

DISTRIBUTORS

USA
Blackwell Mosby Book Distributors
11830 Westline Industrial Drive
St Louis, Missouri 63141

Canada
The C.V. Mosby Company
5240 Finch Avenue East,
Scarborough, Ontario

Australia
Blackwell Scientific Publications
  (Australia) Pty Ltd
107 Barry Street
Carlton, Victoria 3053

British Library
Cataloguing in Publication Data

Ellis, F.R.
  Essential anaesthesia.
  1. Anesthesia
  I. Title II. Campbell, I.T.
  617'.96   RD81

ISBN 0-632-01578-0

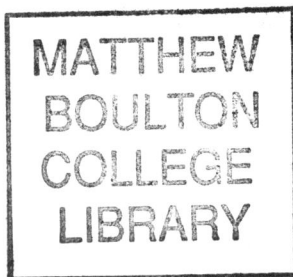

Contents

vi *Contents*

Preface

This short book on anaesthetics and related topics has been written for medical students who are attending a clinical attachment in anaesthesia. Most benefit will be gained if students read the book during the attachment as it will complement but not replace clinical experience gained in the wards, operating theatres, intensive care unit, casualty and out-patient departments. Details of practical procedures have been largely omitted as it is felt the only real way of learning these is by practical demonstration.

Some chapters, such as those on pre-operative preparation and post-operative care, are of vital importance to the student when he becomes a house officer. Others, such as the management of head injury and obstetric analgesia, are covered in other parts of the medical curriculum but usually from a different aspect. This should help the student to get some appreciation of the scope of anaesthesia as a specialty.

We are grateful to our students for their comments and also to a number of our colleagues, namely Drs Tom Bryson, Andy Cohen, Mark Dearden, Tony Nightingale and Freda Roberts.

F.R. ELLIS
I.T. CAMPBELL

Chapter 1

Development of Anaesthesia as a Medical Specialty

Anaesthesia started with a bang in 1846 when William Morton, a Boston dentist, demonstrated the anaesthetic properties of diethylether to a critical surgical audience in Massachusetts General Hospital. The original operating theatre, now known as the Ether Dome, has been preserved. Later the same year nitrous oxide began to be used as an anaesthetic, although it had been inhaled sporadically from 1800 usually on social occasions to induce frolics. In 1847 James Simpson, an Edinburgh obstetrician, first used chloroform.

These events were recognized to be of great importance and soon the demand by surgeons and patients became sufficient for some doctors to be able to devote much of their time to this new branch of medicine. Foremost amongst them was John Snow, who recorded his experiences and eventually wrote a textbook of anaesthesia which was published posthumously. His critical scientific approach did much to develop the new specialty; he was the first specialist anaesthetist. Following John Snow's premature death, Joseph Clover emerged as a thoughtful and innovative pioneer who developed apparatus for the administration of nitrous oxide. He was the first anaesthetist to use an ether–nitrous oxide sequence.

Inhalational anaesthesia was continually modified and refined in the latter part of the century. However, it was some time before oxygen was first added to the anaesthetic mixture (1868) and even up to the early 1960s patients were often allowed to become hypoxic.

Important developments which provided for the necessary skills of modern anaesthesia include the use of the endotracheal tube (Macewen in 1878) and intermittent positive pressure ventilation of the lungs to protect against drug-induced

1

respiratory failure. The invention of the hollow metallic needle and hypodermic syringe (Wood 1853, and Pravaz 1853, respectively) enabled nerve block anaesthesia to be induced with cocaine (Halsted and Corning in 1885), and much later the use of intravenous anaesthesia. Sodium thiopentone (Pentothal) was first used in 1934 by Lundy, although various intravenous agents had been used before this including chloral hydrate from 1875.

Intravenous blood transfusions, so much a part of present day anaesthetic management, have only recently achieved such prominence. Cirtrate for anticoagulation was discovered in 1914 and the classical studies of Landsteiner and Shattock describing the blood groups were published only 14 years earlier.

The full impact of the recognition of the value of curare and its introduction into anaesthetic practice in 1942 by Griffith and Johnson in Montreal was not fully appreciated for over a decade. With hindsight, 1942 was one of the most important 'milestones' in anaesthesia, and provided a rational basis for the current concept of balanced anaesthesia which incorporates unconsciousness, analgesia and muscle relaxation. Until the relaxants were used, muscle paralysis was virtually impossible and relaxation was only achieved with potentially dangerous deep anaesthesia. Over the last 25 years there has been a move towards recognition and maintenance of physiological homeostasis. With better physiological control, anaesthesia has become relatively safe and has allowed the development of cardiac, pulmonary and brain surgery.

It was soon realized that anaesthetists should be involved in the medical management of the unconscious patient due to the need to protect the airway from soiling with gastric contents by the use of endotracheal intubation. Throughout the 1950s and 1960s intensive care units gradually evolved so that patients requiring ventilatory support could be grouped together for better economy of nursing staff, medical time and use of specialized apparatus. These developments marked the beginning of the emergence of the anaesthetist from the narrower confines of the operating theatre.

Most intensive care units are run by anaesthetists because of the common need to control respiration. In this setting the anaesthetist has become more involved with acute post-operative problems, renal failure, head injury, multiple trauma, septic shock, etc. No one doctor can know enough to treat such a wide variety of serious clinical conditions, but the anaesthetist is perhaps better placed than any other doctor to look after the acutely ill patient and to seek expert advice from other specialists such as renal physicians and surgeons. Throughout the last 30 years another branch of anaesthesia has developed, namely, the treatment of pain. In the obstetric field this has led to the development of an epidural analgesia service which complements the traditional methods of pain relief in labour with intravenous agents and inhalational methods with anaesthetic vapours and gases. The problems of intractable pain have broadened the anaesthetist's interests and in most centres pain therapy clinics have been established. Although control of intractable pain concerns many disciplines including general practitioners, psychiatrists and neurosurgeons, the anaesthetist has been able to contribute significantly because of his interest in analgesic drugs and his technical expertise with nerve blocks.

In the modern District General Hospital the anaesthetist contributes to wide-ranging types of treatment and diagnostic procedures. Although his role in the operating theatre remains central to his activities, many anaesthetists spend a greater time in work outside the operating theatre. Anaesthesia is now the largest single hospital-based specialty. It should no longer be thought of as one of the surgical disciplines, but as an independent specialty.

Chapter 2

Principles of General Anaesthesia

Anaesthesia is defined as the absence or abolition of sensation, and should be differentiated from *analgesia* which is the absence or abolition of pain. In the operating theatre the anaesthetist renders the patient free of pain and supports his vital functions — cardiovascular and respiratory systems, cerebral and renal perfusion, etc. — whilst providing satisfactory operating conditions for the surgeon. Anaesthesia that involves rendering the patient unconscious is usually termed general anaesthesia, and anaesthesia provided by blocking conduction in the nerves either in, or supplying, the operation site is termed local anaesthesia (or analgesia.)

In addition to analgesia, the surgeon often requires muscle relaxation to allow him to operate. The degree of relaxation required depends on the operation but is greatest with upper abdominal surgery. From the introduction of general anaesthesia as a technique until the development of muscle relaxants, the three requirements of sleep, analgesia and muscle relaxation were achieved using one drug. This was unsatisfactory, because if enough of the drug were given to produce adequate muscle relaxation, depression of the cardiovascular and respiratory systems occurred due to the drug's depressant action on the cardiovascular and respiratory centres in the medulla. Most general anaesthetic agents have other undesirable side effects as well, and these include flammability, nausea and vomiting, stimulation of salivary and bronchial secretions, sensitization of the myocardium to circulating catecholamines and direct myocardial depression.

INHALATIONAL INDUCTION OF ANAESTHESIA

General anaesthesia was originally induced by an ether or chloroform-soaked silk handkerchief (or piece of lint) placed over the face. Room air was inhaled through the material thus vaporizing the agent which passed with the inspired air into the lungs and then to the brain. Using this technique of induction with ether, the depth of anaesthesia achieved was described and classified into four stages. The characteristics of the different stages vary slightly with other agents, but still follow the same basic pattern.

Stage I: Analgesia

The patient is conscious and rational, but perception of pain is diminished.

Stage II: Confusion, excitement or delirium

The most dangerous stage. The patient is unconscious but responds reflexly and irrationally to stimuli and may be violent; breath holding may result in hypoxia and he may vomit. Tone is still present in the pharyngeal muscles, so he is, in theory, capable of maintaining his own airway. Laryngeal and respiratory reflexes are retained, so if the patient does vomit, soiling of the respiratory tract is usually accompanied by coughing, laryngeal spasm, etc.

Stage III: Surgical anaesthesia

The stage at which surgery can take place. Increasing depth of anaesthesia within this stage is associated with increasing degrees of muscle relaxation. Protective pharyngotracheal reflexes are absent and he is unable to maintain his own airway. Any reflux of stomach contents is due to passive regurgitation, and soiling of the respiratory tract is not associated with reflex coughing or laryngeal spasm, and so may go unnoticed until respiratory distress develops later.

Stage IV: Medullary depression

Cardiovascular and respiratory failure occur as a result of depression of the cardiovascular and respiratory centres in the medulla.

SIGNS OF ANAESTHETIC DEPTH

With 'rag and bottle' anaesthesia it was possible to tell how deeply anaesthetized a patient was, in relation to the scheme outlined above, by observing changes occurring in the respiratory pattern, in the eyes and pupils, and in the response to stimuli. These changes are still relevant to modern anaesthetic practice, especially in spontaneously breathing patients.

Respiration

Stage I — normal. Expiration is longer than inspiration with the occasional sigh. In Stage II breathing is often irregular and can be associated with breath holding. Stage III is heralded by the onset of a respiratory pattern very regular both in rhythm and in depth; the expiratory phase is shortened and tends to equal inspiration. As Stage III deepens respiration is steadily depressed, with greater depression of the intercostal muscles than of the diaphragm. In Stage IV respiration ceases as a result of central depression.

Pupils

Pupillary changes depend on the drug. Ether dilates the pupils but most other agents constrict them and drugs given at the same time, such as morphine and atropine, have their own specific effects. In Stage II and the early part of Stage III, the pupils react to light and the eyeballs may be eccentric becoming central again as anaesthesia deepens.

Response to stimuli

There is an active response to stimuli in Stages I and II, in Stage I rationally, and in Stage II reflexly or irrationally. Stimuli tend to arouse and if the patient is lightly anaesthetized in Stage III this may move him into Stage II which could be hazardous.

UPTAKE OF INHALATIONAL ANAESTHETIC AGENTS

Inhalational anaesthetic agents act on the brain. They get there via the inspired gases, the alveoli, the pulmonary capillary, pulmonary venous and systemic arterial blood. The rate of induction of anaesthesia is determined by the rate at which the partial pressure of the agent in the brain approaches that in the inspired gas. During stable anaesthesia the gradient between the partial pressure in the alveoli and the partial pressure in the brain is small, there being a huge area of alveolar capillary membrane taking part in gas exchange, and the brain is well supplied with blood. In the resting individual the brain receives about 15% of cardiac output. The partial pressure of the agent in the alveoli therefore closely reflects the partial pressure of the agent in the brain. The factors that affect the rate of increase of partial pressure in the brain, and thus the rate of induction of anaesthesia, are therefore the same as those which affect the rate of increase of partial pressure in the alveoli. These are:

1 *Inspired concentration.*

2 *Alveolar ventilation.*

3 *Solubility.* The more soluble an anaesthetic agent (e.g. trichlorethylene) the more readily it is taken up by the tissues, the more slowly alveolar (and brain) partial pressure increases and the more slowly the patient goes to sleep. The less soluble the agent is (e.g. cyclopropane) the more rapidly does alveolar concentration rise and the more rapid is induction.

4 *Cardiac output.* A high cardiac output will mop up large quantities of anaesthetic agent from the alveoli, and the alveolar concentration will rise slowly; induction will therefore be slow. The paradox of higher uptakes of the agent associated with a slower rate of induction is due to the fact that a high cardiac output is normally caused by the patient struggling, so most of the increased output (and uptake) goes to skeletal muscle. At the other extreme, in a patient with low cardiac output due, for example, to blood loss, relatively little of the agent is taken up, alveolar concentration rises rapidly and induction is rapid. In this instance a much higher proportion of the total cardiac output goes to the brain. For this reason, hypovolaemic patients are very sensitive to anaesthetic agents.

MINIMUM ALVEOLAR CONCENTRATION

Minimum alveolar concentration (MAC) is an index of the potency of an inhalational anaesthetic agent. It is defined in clinical terms as the alveolar concentration at which half the patients do not move in response to a surgical stimulus. There is a rough correlation between the MAC value of an inhalational anaesthetic agent and its lipid solubility.

THE 'TRIAD OF ANAESTHESIA'

The introduction of muscle relaxants revolutionized anaesthesia and surgery. Muscle relaxation could be produced with a neuromuscular blocking drug, such as tubocurarine, the patient could be put to sleep with an intravenous induction agent, such as sodium thiopentone, analgesia produced with an intravenous analgesic such as morphine, and sleep maintained with nitrous oxide only or with minimal concentrations of an inhalational agent. *Sleep, analgesia* and *muscle relaxation* represent the so-called *triad of anaesthesia*.

Paralysis of all skeletal muscles by neuromuscular blockade will include the respiratory muscles, so respiration ceases. At about the time neuromuscular blocking agents were introduced into clinical practice, the technique of intermittent positive pressure ventilation (IPPV) was devised, whereby the lung is ventilated by the intermittent application of a flow of fresh gas to the airway under positive pressure. At its simplest, this was achieved by squeezing, by hand, a rebreathing bag attached to the patient's airway. Over the years this technique has been developed and refined and its use extended beyond the operating theatre, leading ultimately to the development of surgical and respiratory intensive care units.

Reversal of the neuromuscular blockade produced by tubocurarine is by means of an anticholinesterase drug, usually neostigmine. This blocks choline esterase, the enzyme that destroys acetylcholine. Acteylcholine concentrations around the motor end plate increase, and displace tubocurarine from the end plate, and recovery of neuromuscular transmission takes place.

GAS EXCHANGE AND ANAESTHETIC CIRCUITRY

On induction of anaesthesia a number of changes occur in the patient's cardiovascular and respiratory physiology which affect gas exchange in the lung. Ventilation/perfusion relationships are disturbed and alterations take place in cardiac output. Respiratory dead space increases. The ultimate outcome is a decrease in the efficiency of gas exchange in the lung with an increase in pulmonary 'shunting' and a tendency to hypoxaemia. If respiratory depression takes place, not only is the hypoxaemia worse but carbon dioxide retention occurs as well. It is the anaesthetist's responsibility to avoid carbon dioxide retention and hypoxia. Because of the increase in pulmonary shunt this means that any anaesthetized patient must have an inspired oxygen concentration of at least 30%. Any apparatus used to deliver anaesthetic gases to a patient must be designed so that:

1 predictable concentrations of oxygen and anaesthetic vapour can be delivered, and

2 the CO_2 produced is eliminated from the circuit.

A number of anaesthetic circuits are in common use. All are designed with these principles in mind. It is your responsibility to acquaint yourself with the characteristics of the circuits in use in your own hospital.

Chapter 3

Pharmacology of Drugs Used in Anaesthesia

INHALATIONAL AGENTS

Vapours

Halothane for many years has been the most commonly used supplement to nitrous oxide anaesthesia throughout the world. It was synthesized by ICI Pharmaceuticals plc and introduced into clinical practice in 1956. It is a comparatively stable, non-inflammable, easily volatized fluid, with a boiling point (b.p.) of 50°C. Halothane is a potent anaesthetic with poor direct analgesia properties (characteristics which therefore perfectly complement nitrous oxide). The drug acts directly on the heart, reducing cardiac output, and on blood vessels, causing vasodilatation and hypotension. An increase in vagal tone causes bradycardia. The uterus will relax in deep halothane obstetric anaesthesia, resulting in postpartum haemorrhage. Halothane depresses respiration centrally, though respiratory rate may increase due to activation of peripheral reflexes by the irritant vapour. The two major complications are halothane hepatitis and malignant hyperpyrexia (see Chapter 11).

Diethyl ether, usually simply referred to as ether, has remained a safe and popular anaesthetic for many years. It is still commonly used in Third World countries. Ether has a lower b.p. (35°C) than halothane, but due to its greater solubility in blood is a slower induction agent. The major problem with ether is its flammability in air and its explosive properties with oxygen and with nitrous oxide/oxygen gas mixtures. Ether anaesthesia has a wide safety margin, as respiratory failure occurs only with very deep anaesthesia. Its major advantages include pronounced analgesia and skeletal muscle relaxation. It

10

increases circulating catecholamines due to central stimulation. Post-operatively many patients vomit and most patients complain of the persistent unpleasant taste which lasts for many hours. Post-operative recovery may be prolonged due to its great solubility in tissue fluids.

Chloroform has not been used widely for many years as it causes both liver damage and heart failure in an unpredictable manner.

Enflurane (Ethrane) is one of the newer halogen substituted non-inflammable ethers. As an ether it has better analgesic properties than halothane but otherwise is little different in use.

Trichloroethylene is still used as a supplement to nitrous oxide during short procedures. It has a high b.p. of 87°C and though a potent anaesthetic is difficult to use due to problems with vaporization. It is a powerful analgesic in low concentrations and can be used with air for obstetric analgesia. In presentation it has a blue colour owing to the addition of the dye waxolene blue. It must never be used in closed circuits as the nerve gas phosgene can be produced with soda lime.

Methoxyflurane is not now recommended for clinical use as it can induce renal failure. As an ether it was a powerful analgesic and was used in midwifery.

Gases

Nitrous oxide at normal ambient temperatures is stored as a liquid in cylinders at 50 atmospheres, the cylinder pressure only falling when the liquid has evaporated completely. It is a weak anaesthetic but a powerful analgesic. Its pharmacological actions are of a rapid onset due to the rapid rise of PN_2O in the blood due to its comparative insolubility; 100 ml of blood can only dissolve 47 ml N_2O. The main danger is hypoxia due to the inadvertent exclusion of oxygen. Nitrous oxide has little significant effect on cardiovascular or respiratory systems though prolonged use results in bone marrow depression. At the end of a long nitrous oxide anaesthetic, the mass movement of the gas from the body tissues into the alveolar gas can cause the alveolar Po_2 to fall precipitously causing diffusion hypoxia.

Entonox is a 50:50 mixture of nitrous oxide and oxygen. As an analgesic it is used both in the ambulance service and in obstetrics by non-medical staff. Efficient use of Entonox results in effective oxygen therapy and so should be used with care in chronic lung disease.

Cyclopropane is little used due to the danger of explosion. It is a powerful anaesthetic with a very rapid induction, and can be helpful when intravenous (i.v.) anaesthesia is difficult (e.g. in paediatrics) or is contra-indicated such as with severe heart disease.

Oxygen is stored at 132 atmospheres. The cylinder outlet must be kept free of oil or grease which can ignite at high pressure (as in a diesel engine). Anaesthetized patients should always receive at least 21% oxygen, but preferably over 30%.

Carbon dioxide is to be found on most British anaesthetic machines and is used usually to stimulate respiration which is depressed due to hypocapnia following prolonged artificial ventilation of the lungs. If CO_2 is administered to a normocapnic individual, respiration is stimulated, cerebral blood flow increased and thus inhalational anaesthetic drugs will act more rapidly on the brain. Blind intubation of the trachea is also easier as the glottis widens during inspiration as hypercapnoia is induced.

A *helium and oxygen* (80:20) gas mixture has a much lower density than air and is used to oxygenate patients with severe partial airway obstruction which cannot be relieved simply.

INTRAVENOUS INDUCTION AGENTS

Thiopentone (Pentothal), a thiobarbiturate, has been used since 1934 and is still the most popular i.v. induction drug. It is fairly unstable in solution and needs to be freshly dissolved in water to make a highly alkaline solution which also contains sodium carbonate. A 2.5% solution is used, as 5% has caused gangrene when injected intra-arterially by mistake. On i.v. injection a dose of around 3 mg per kg produces anaesthesia within one arm–brain circulation time. Respiratory depression (after a brief stimulation) is usual and apnoea can last for up to 30 seconds. When respiration returns it is of reduced depth rather than rate. The contractability of the heart is reduced and the cardiac output falls. Blood pressure (BP) falls due to peripheral vasodilatation and venous pooling. Rarely laryngeal or bronchial spasm occurs. The acute effects of thiopentone terminate with its redistribution; its complete breakdown occurs over several hours in the liver and the metabolites are excreted by the kidneys. Thiopentone is a good anticonvulsant and it depresses the sympathetic nervous system centrally. It should be used with care in all cases of heart disease, and should never be given to patients with porphyria who can develop an exacerbation of the disease with demyelination.

Methohexitone (Brietal) is an oxybarbiturate which is almost three times as potent as thiopentone. More muscle movements are seen than with thiopentone. This drug is used for short procedures in out-patients as recovery is minimally quicker.

Several other drugs have been introduced in the last decade. One of the main aims has been to avoid barbiturates which, being slowly metabolized, cause prolonged drowsiness. All recently introduced drugs are rapidly metabolized. Propanidid, derived from oil of cloves, requires a solubilising agent cremorph. Propanidid has caused anaphylactic reactions and has been largely replaced, first by Althesin, a mixture of two steroids with similar allergenic problems, and later by etomidate, an imidazole derivative. Etomidate has been shown to reduce cortisol levels when used as an infusion for prolonged periods but the significance of this is not fully understood. It can produce pain on injection and thrombophlebitis.

Ketamine (Ketalar) is an interesting drug related to phencyclidine which causes bizarre hallucinations. Ketamine produces a dissociative anaesthesia. It is a good analgesic which causes a rise in BP and tachycardia due to a rise in plasma catecholamines. Respiration is not depressed and the protective reflexes are not obtunded. Its main use is in children, for multiple anaesthetics (e.g. burns dressings) and in situations where anaesthetists are unavailable.

ANALGESICS

Major opiates and opioids

Morphine is our best tried and most reliable analgesic with a history of over 2000 years. It is usually given by intramuscular (i.m.) injection and its oral potency is about half that of parenteral administration. Morphine depresses respiration in relation to its analgesic action, and depresses cerebrocortical activity, producing euphoria and relief from anxiety. Its main drawbacks are its tendency to induce nausea and vomiting by a central action, its depressive action on gut which causes constipation, and its tendency to release histamine which makes it a potentially dangerous drug for asthmatics.

Diamophine (Heroin) is twice as potent as morphine and as it is much more soluble it can be administered in a small volume. This makes it particularly suitable for the terminally sick and cachexic patient.

Papaveretum (Omnopon) contains several opiates though its most important ingredient is morphine. It has an equivalent potency of 65% of morphine.

Pethidine was one of the first synthetic opioids. Its main advantage is to relax smooth muscle and it is therefore indicated in renal and biliary colic, and to relax bronchospasm. It has atropine-like actions producing tachycardia and a dry mouth, and in some individuals causes marked hypotension, sweating and sickness.

Fentanyl (and *phenoperidine*) is related to pethidine chemically but is roughly 1000 times more potent. It has a marked respiratory depressive action but causes little effect on the cardiovascular system. Fentanyl has been used for i.v. induction of anaesthesia in patients with severe cardiovascular disease. The analgesic properties of fentanyl last for 30–45 minutes and those of phenoperidine for twice as long. *Alfentanil* is a new drug which has a shorter duration and may find a place in out-patients anaesthesia.

Narcotic antagonists

These drugs compete for cell membrane receptors as they are n-allyl derivatives of opiates.

Naloxone has no analgesic activity and is used to reverse opioid respiratory depression.

Nalorphine and *levallorphan* have some agonist activity and should be administered while carefully monitoring their effect.

Minor opiates and opioids

Codeine phosphate and *dihydrocodeine* (DF118) have similar properties to the major opiates except without respiratory depression and nausea, but are considerably less potent as analgesics. Although central effects are minimal, patients can become addicted when receiving these drugs for chronic pain.

Pentazocine (Fortral) has a mild opioid antagonist property and will tend to reverse opioid respiratory depression but can induce hallucinations.

Buprenorphine (Temgesic) is a much more powerful narcotic antagonist and should not be combined with opioids. It has a prolonged action. Buprenorphine can be administered as a sublingual tablet which is rapidly effective, though often causes sickness in the ambulant patient.

This group of drugs is rapidly expanding in numbers with special claims made for the new arrivals. Advantages would include lack of additive properties, no respiratory depression, no associated nausea and no constipation.

ANTICHOLINERGICS

Atropine has two main uses. As a premedicant drug it acts as an antisialogogue particularly with a drug such as ether which causes copious secretions to be produced. Its most important action is as an antivagal drug which protects the heart from reflex bradycardia induced by a variety of drugs including anticholinesterases during reversal of non-depolarizing relaxants. It also has some anti-emetic properties due to both central and peripheral mechanisms by a direct action on the emetic centre and by reducing bowel activity. It inhibits the cholinergic sympathetic fibres responsible for sweating and thus can cause a rise in body temperature by abolishing one of the important heat loss mechanisms.

Hyoscine (Scopolamine) is an alternative drug to atropine as a premedicant and has the advantage of more sedation and some amnesia. Old patients do not tolerate hyoscine well even though the action on the heart is less pronounced than with atropine. Hyoscine is not used during relaxant reversal.

Glycopyrrolate has been introduced as an alternative to atropine. It has a greater duration of action without central effects as it does not cross the blood–brain barrier.

MUSCLE RELAXANTS

The muscle relaxants are drugs which act on the post-junctional receptors at the neuromuscular junction, and are divided into two separate groups based on pharmacological characteristics. The depolarizers act by depolarizing the post-synaptic membrane and causing paralysis by inhibiting the restoration of the normal membrane polarity. They are partial agonists for acetylcholine, have slender molecules, and initially activate muscle causing muscle fasciculations, liberation of potassium and myoglobin, and they often produce muscle pains postoperatively. The non-depolarizers have elaborate molecules, compete with acetylcholine receptors and stabilize the post-synaptic membrane.

Suxamethonium (Succinyldicholine, Scoline) is the only depolarizer in common use. As a partial agonist it causes muscle fasciculation, and a rise in both serum potassium and CK due to muscle damage. Post-operatively around 30% of patients experience muscle pain in the muscles of the shoulder girdle and intercostals; these pains can mimic pleurisy. A first or a second dose of suxamethonium can cause a potentially dangerous bradycardia due to vagotonic effects which can be prevented by atropine. The muscle relaxation with suxamethonium is of rapid onset and lasts 3–5 minutes and it is terminated rapidly by esteratic cleavage of the molecule with plasma cholinesterase. These characteristics make it an ideal drug for tracheal intubation. Two major problems with suxamethonium are an inherited deficiency of the plasma cholinesterase causing prolonged apnoea ('Scoline apnoea'), and malignant hyperpyrexia. Predisposition to both conditions is inherited as recessive and as dominant characteristics respectively.

(+) *Tubocurarine* (Curare, derived from South American arrow poison) acts as an acetylcholine competitor, thus preventing end-plate activation. Muscles of the face are paralysed before those of the abdominal wall and diaphragm. Curare lasts 30–60 minutes although the duration is dose-dependent. High doses cause hypotension due to autonomic ganglionic blockade and histamine can be liberated. Thirty per cent is excreted unchanged by the kidneys.

Pancuronium has a steroid molecule as its foundation, though without steroid activity. In use it closely resembles +-tubocurarine although it tends to cause a mild temporary hypertension and it is partially metabolized in the liver and excreted in the bile.

Gallamine and *alcuronium* are shorter-acting non-depolarizers which still have a place in clinical anaesthesia for medium length operations.

Atracurium and *vecuronium* are exciting new additions to the non-depolarizers. Both drugs are of rapid onset and short duration and can be used as alternatives to suxamethonium under certain circumstances without the undisputed dangers of suxamethonium. Also, being non-depolarizers, they can be reversed with anticholinesterases. Atracurium has already been shown to be valuable for anephric patients who have problems with other relaxants and undergoes spontaneous degradation in the body.

ANTICHOLINESTERASES

Neostigmine (Prostigmine) prevents the hydrolysis of acetylcholine by cholinesterase and the resulting accumulation of acetylcholine dislodges the non-depolarizer molecule from the acetylcholine receptor. Neostigmine causes dangerous bradycardia unless combined with atropine. If given in large dosage, neostigmine can result in a depolarizing block due to excessive acetylcholine. The muscarinic properties of neostigmine cause increased bowel activity which could endanger surgical bowel anastomosis, increase secretions and cause bronchoconstriction.

Edrophonium (Tensilon) is a much shorter-acting drug than neostigmine and so is used to test the need for further anticholinesterase when relaxant reversal is inadequate, and also to test for myasthenia gravis.

TRANQUILLIZERS, ANXIOLYTICS AND NEUROLEPTICS

The *phenothiazines* are important drugs as they have many useful properties including sedation and removal of anxiety, inhibition of the central sympathetic nervous sytem, depression of the temperature regulating centre in the hypothalamus, reduction of blood pressure by both central and peripheral mechanisms, anti-emesis and inhibition of shivering. Prochlorperazine (Stemetil) is used as an anti-emetic, trimeprazine (Vallergan) is a valuable premedicant for small children, as is promethazine (Phenergan) for adults. Chlorpromazine (Largactil) has been used as an anti-adrenaline drug and to inhibit shivering.

Diazepam, the most used benzodiazepine, is a valuable drug as an anxiolytic for premedication and also during local anaesthetic procedures. A combination of diazepam and lipids (Diazemuls) is less painful on i.v. administration. Rarely, diazepam causes respiratory insufficiency and cardiovascular collapse, especially in the elderly. It is not analgesic but is an effective anticonvulsant and controls abnormal drug-induced muscle movements.

Droperidol is a butyrophenone which causes mental detachment and is used in neuroleptanalgesia with a potent analgesic such as fentanyl. It is also a weak alpha-adrenaline blocker and a good anti-emetic which specifically inhibits the chemoreceptor trigger zone. It has a long duration and may increase anxiety due to inability to communicate.

Chapter 4

Pre-Operative Assessment

Death due to anaesthesia alone is now rare. The morbidity and mortality of surgery are due to factors present before, during and after operation. These include blood loss, tissue damage, enforced fasting, immobility, pain and hypoxia. The statement that a patient is 'fit for anaesthesia' is now meaningless.

When a patient with an intercurrent illness presents for surgery three factors have to be considered:
1 the nature, the extent and the urgency of the operation;
2 the effect of the operation and its associated morbidity on the patient's homeostatic mechanisms; and
3 the effect of anaesthesia.

The nature of the anaesthetic must be decided upon in the light of factors 1 and 2. It would for example be wiser to repair a hernia in an unstable insulin-dependent diabetic under some form of local anaesthetic than under general anaesthesia. This would allow him to resume oral intake and insulin injections earlier than otherwise. The mortality of surgery and anaesthesia for a bleeding peptic ulcer is improved if the patient is resuscitated prior to surgery, but it would be unwise to spend a prolonged period attempting to resuscitate a patient bleeding from a ruptured ectopic pregnancy or a bleeding aortic aneurysm. The dangers of elective surgery for a peptic ulcer in a man with severe coronary artery disease and a history of recent myocardial infarction has to be weighed against the chances that his ulcer may bleed or may perforate. If a decision is taken against elective operation and the ulcer does perforate, he will then have to be operated on as an emergency in a much poorer condition than if the operation had been done electively.

ASSESSMENT OF FITNESS FOR SURGERY

An assessment of a patient's general condition is provided by the American Society of Anesthesiologists Physical Status Scale. This rates a patient's general condition on a grading of 1–5 as follows:

Grade 1   A normal healthy individual
Grade 2   A patient with a systemic disease but no functional impairment
Grade 3   A patient with a systemic disease and significant functional impairment
Grade 4   A patient with a systemic disease and severe impairment of function
Grade 5   A moribund patient not expected to survive more than 24 hours with or without operation.

This is a pre-operative assessment scale and does not predict surgical outcome, though the two are obviously indirectly related.

In normal circumstances the house surgeon has seen the patient, taken a full medical history and carried out a full physical examination. If he elicits facts which he is aware may concern the anaesthetist, he should alert him to his findings so that the patient can be assessed in plenty of time and any necessary investigations and/or treatment instituted prior to operation.

All patients should be routinely seen by an anaesthetist the night before surgery and ideally by the person going to administer the anaesthetic. A formal medical history and a full physical examination is, in most instances, not necessary, but a series of specific leading questions should be asked along the following lines.

Previous anaesthetics and operations

Questions about previous anaesthetics may reveal incidents such as a period of prolonged vomiting after a previous operation, or prolonged apnoea after suxamethonium administration or a previous operation which affects anaesthetic management such as a cervical fusion. Anaesthetic family history could reveal a family trait for plasma cholinesterase deficiency or malignant hyperpyrexia.

Medical illness

Patients should be specifically asked if they suffer from diseases of heart, chest, liver, kidney or nervous system. The assessment and significance of chest and heart disease will be discussed later in this chapter. Some of the other conditions which commonly affect anaesthesia and surgery are discussed in Chapter 7.

Drugs

Patients should be asked if they take drugs regularly. Having denied any illnesses a patient may, on occasion, admit to taking hypotensive agents or anti-epileptic drugs. He may have been living with his condition for so long that he has ceased to regard it as an illness.

Drug allergy

This must be asked for and documented.

Smoking and drinking habits

A high alcohol intake raises the possibility of liver disease and tends to be associated with a relative insensitivity to anaesthetic and analgesic drugs. Heavy smoking is associated with chronic bronchitis and respiratory function should be assessed.

Local problems

Difficulties in maintaining the airway or problems with intubation can often be anticipated from the pre-operative visit and appropriate precautions taken. Obesity and the absence of teeth often cause airway problems, and a small mouth, a high arched palate, receding chin, very prominent teeth and an inability to open the mouth properly are all findings which are associated with intubation difficulties.

Physical examination

This is routinely directed to the respiratory and cardiovascular systems but should be extended to other systems or parts of the body if there are indications to do so (e.g. osteoarthritis of the hips in a patient who will be in the lithotomy position). Specific attention should be paid, particularly in emergencies, to the state of hydration, including urine output, and, if necessary, should be corrected with intravenous fluids before operation.

PRE-OPERATIVE LABORATORY AND RADIOLOGICAL INVESTIGATIONS

Investigations such as ECG, chest X-ray, etc. are performed to supplement the pre-operative history and examination for three reasons:

1 as a means of assessing the severity of a known condition;
2 as a normal base line in case complications occur during or after operation; and
3 as a screening procedure for an otherwise apparently healthy population, although in times of financial stringency it is doubtful if this is justified.

As a general rule the routine investigations required for any patient undergoing surgery are as follows:

1 *The haemoglobin concentration.* It is generally considered desirable that this should be in excess of 10 gm/100 ml.
2 *Urine testing* may identify the occasional patient suffering from previously unsuspected diabetes or renal disease.

For patients undergoing major surgery, particularly those over the age of 40, the following investigations should also be done:

3 *Electrolytes and urea.* Normal cellular function depends on electrolyte concentrations in intra and extra cellular fluid and on acid base status. If these are abnormal pre-operatively the response to anaesthetic drugs and the trauma of surgery will be impaired. The response to muscle relaxants is also abnormal in the presence of electrolyte or acid base disturbances and difficulties may arise in reversing these drugs after the operation.
4 *Chest X-ray* helps in the assessment of chest disease and shows up cardiac enlargement or early pulmonary oedema. It is useful for comparison if chest complications arise post-operatively.
5 *The ECG* may show previously unsuspected heart disease, particularly in older patients, and helps in the assessment of patients with known heart disease. Again it is a base line if abnormalities are noted during or after the operation.

6 *In some types of surgery blood transfusion is nearly always required,* e.g. aortic surgery, extensive bowel resections, etc., so blood should be routinely cross-matched. In others such as cholecstectomy, vagotomy and pyloroplasty, thyroidectomy, injection of oesophageal varices, etc., it is not normally needed, but if complications arise or unexpected pathology is found requiring more extensive surgery, blood transfusion may be necessary. For operations such as these blood is usually taken, the patient's blood group determined pre-operatively and the serum is then saved for cross-matching if blood is needed.

CARDIORESPIRATORY FUNCTION

Signs and symptoms of the cardiovascular and respiratory systems frequently overlap: exertional dyspnoea, orthopnoea, cough, etc. The history, physical examination and laboratory investigations help determine where the primary pathology lies, but in terms of function and response to operation the two systems can be considered together. The best way to judge this at the bedside is in terms of exercise tolerance. If a patient gives a reliable history of being able to climb a flight of stairs with no difficulty, problems are unlikely to occur. If the history is in doubt he should be made to do so and observed. With an exercise tolerance less than this the likelihood of problems arising increases.

Respiratory disease

The immobility and the impaired ability to cough or breath deeply with an abdominal wound may cause an upper respiratory tract infection to develop into bronchopneumonia. As a general rule patients with a common cold presenting for elective surgery should be postponed. Patients with chronic chest disease should have their condition improved as much as possible prior to surgery. This means:
1 *Sputum culture* and, if necessary, a pre-operative course of antibiotics.
2 *Physiotherapy* and deep breathing exercises which should be continued post-operatively.
3 *Bronchodilators* if necessary.
4 *Respiratory Function Tests* performed pre-operatively give an objective indication of the severity of respiratory disease.

The simplest, most commonly performed tests are measurements of:

the forced votal capacity (FVC) — a measure of lung volume

the forced expiratory volume in 1 second (FEV_1) and

the ratio FEV_1/FVC — an index of airways obstruction

These measurements compared with the values predicted for age, sex, height and weight indicate the severity of respiratory disease, but are only an adjunct to the history and physical examination.

The patients with respiratory disease who have the most problems after operation, perhaps requiring a period of intermittent positive pressure ventilation are those whose arterial blood gases are abnormal pre-operatively (i.e. a low Pao_2 and a high $Paco_2$). Arterial gases and acid base status should be measured pre-operatively in patients with severe respiratory disease having a major operation.

Cardiovascular disease

Heart failure

This must be treated prior to surgery with digoxin, diuretics, etc. Many drugs used in anaesthesia produce myocardial depression directly or indirectly and induction of anaesthesia can precipitate overt heart failure.

Recent myocardial infarction

Recent myocardial infarction, i.e. within the preceding 6 months, is associated with a high incidence of re-infarction. The mortality of myocardial infarction in the peri-operative period is also high — in the region of 50%. Risk of re-infarction decreases with time, until 1 or 2 years after the infarction it is no greater than in a normal population. Elective surgery in a patient with a history of recent myocardial infarction should be postponed for as long as reasonably possible.

Hypertension

The dangers of operating on untreated hypertensive patients are the wide swings in blood pressure, particularly severe hypertension, in response to stimuli such as pain or laryngoscopy and endotracheal intubation. The dangers are of cerebrovascular accident, cerebral oedema, pulmonary oedema, myocardial infarction and myocardial ischaemia secondary to the increase in peripheral vascular resistance and the increase in work (after load) that the heart of a hypertensive patient has to do. No patient with severe hypertension should undergo elective surgery until effective treatment has been instituted. The possibility of impaired renal function should also be considered.

Coronary artery disease

The dangers of operating on patients with coronary artery disease and angina are myocardial infarction and myocardial ischaemia. These are particularly dangerous if wide variations in blood pressure, or heart rate, are allowed to occur.

Drug therapy

Several drugs taken for cardiovascular disease affect the cardiovascular responses to anaesthesia and surgery.

Digoxin and diuretics. Serum electrolyte levels must be checked pre-operatively because of the danger of hypokalaemia.

Beta-blockers impair the ability of the cardiac output to change in response to variations in demand. They decrease myocardial contractility and can precipitate heart failure in those patients already on the verge of it. In addition they predispose to bronchospasm. However, the dangers of stopping beta-blockers prior to surgery — cardiac arrythmias, uncontrolled angina and hypertension — are greater than the dangers of continuing them, so in general patients taking beta-blockers should continue to take them and the possible complications of bronchospasm, hypotension, low cardiac output or overt heart failure should be borne in mind. If necessary the cardiac output of a beta-blocked patient can be increased with a competitive beta-agonist such as isoprenaline.

Hypotensive therapy. Patients on antihypertensive agents acting on the peripheral circulation may lose the ability to compensate for decreases in cardiac output caused by blood loss or drugs. It was once considered advisable to stop these prior to surgery, but the dangers of doing so proved to be greater than the benefits, the dangers being uncontrolled swings in blood pressure and the danger of myocardial or cerebral damage. It is now normal practice to continue with hypotensive therapy throughout the peri-operative period.

PREPARATION OF THE PATIENT FOR SURGERY

Fasting

Because of the dangers of vomiting and inhalation of stomach contents during induction, it has become routine practice that every patient is starved to ensure an empty stomach prior to surgery. For a patient having elective surgery on a morning list this means starving from at least midnight the night before. Patients operated on in the afternoons are usually allowed a light breakfast early in the morning (about 6.30 a.m.) but nothing by mouth after that. The problems of routine overnight starvation are hypoglycaemia and dehydration. These are not problems in fit healthy adults but may be in children, or diabetics, or patients with liver disease. Appropriate precautions should be considered, such as intravenous administration of glucose. In young children it is common practice to allow feeds of dextrose and water up to 4 hours pre-operatively.

For emergency surgery the patient should have nothing by mouth for 4 hours pre-operatively although this has to be weighed against the urgency of the surgery. It cannot be guaranteed that any patient has an empty stomach even after an overnight fast. Accident victims often have delayed gastric emptying times. In patients known to have a full stomach, such as those with intestinal obstruction, it is normal practice to pass a nasogastric tube and aspirate the stomach pre-operatively, although it can never be assumed that this is 100% effective. The presence of a nasogastric tube also makes the gastro-oesophageal junction incompetent so the anaesthetist may remove the tube before induction and replace it once the patient is asleep and the airway secure with an endotracheal tube. With any emergency surgery it is wise to assume that the patient's stomach is not empty and to take the appropriate precautions against regurgitation and inhalation of stomach contents, particularly on induction and recovery.

Chapter 5

Premedication

The aims of premedication are:
1 to reduce anxiety and induce euphoria and sedation;
2 to reduce vagal reflexes and so reduce secretions and protect against bradycardia;
3 to provide operative and post-operative analgesia;
4 to reduce anaesthetic requirements.

Anxiety which is experienced by all patients pre-operatively can best be assessed during the anaesthetist's pre-operative visit. Specific anxiolytics such as diazepam are commonly used.

Vagolytic agents including atropine and hyoscine are used less nowadays as premedicants. The anaesthetic drugs in common use, unlike ether, do not cause excessive secretions, and if dangerous parasympathetic reflexes are envisaged, atropine can be given intravenously concurrently. Atropine is more effective than hyoscine to obtund vagal reflexes but hyoscine has the advantages of being sedative and more anti-emetic.

Analgesia is rarely required pre-operatively and the use of opiates is largely to provide an analgesic background for the post-operative period; the peak analgesia after intramuscular morphine is around 2 hours. Premedicant opiates reduce the need for operative opiates with which they summate.

COMMONLY USED PREMEDICATION

Morphine and atropine, papaveretum and hyoscine (Omnopon and Scopolamine), pethidine and atropine are all commonly used combinations especially for major surgery. Pethidine is often given to old patients as it is less depressant.

Diazepam or other benzodiazepine is especially useful for minor surgery when post-operative pain is not anticipated, and it is as effective orally as intramuscularly if given $\frac{1}{2}$–2 hours before anaesthesia. Various combinations of drug are used for specific types of patient or surgery. Promethazine is useful in chronic bronchitics as a bronchodilator. Barbiturates are used for epileptics but these drugs increase post-operative restlessness especially if pain is experienced due to their antanalgesic properties. Droperidol has been used as a sedative agent especially for patients for whom neuroleptanaesthesia is planned; however, its neuroleptic properties are far from ideal and are shown to increase anxiety.

Hypnotics are often administered the night before surgery to help with sleep which is often disturbed in the unfamiliar surroundings of a hospital ward. The most useful drugs are found to include chloral hydrate, nitrazepam, barbiturates and some phenothiazines.

Chapter 6

Care of the Unconscious

Although the anaesthetized subject is unconscious, this chapter is concerned not with the care of the anaesthetized so much as with the management of unconsciousness from other causes, including disease or poisoning of and trauma to the brain. As the unconscious state may continue for days, months and even years, it is important to try to establish a working prognosis at the outset before irreversible decisions have been made, such as whether to ventilate the lungs mechanically. If maximal support of bodily functions is undertaken, a vegetative state can be prolonged almost indefinitely. A decision concerning whether to treat actively must be taken by someone with experience, as in practice it becomes very difficult to revert to a less active treatment. Although there are many 'grey' areas, such as hepatic failure, it is generally accepted that unconsciousness secondary to malignant disease is usually best left untreated and the patient allowed to die without active support of bodily functions.

THE LUNGS

The management of the respiratory system depends on the ability of the patient to spontaneously ventilate adequately, and whether the protective reflexes are normally active.

The most urgent problem in the unconscious is to ensure an adequate airway due to the loss of the ability to protrude the tongue; impaction of the tongue in the posterior pharynx is the commonest cause of airway obstruction. Signs of airway obstruction include:
1 cyanosis when breathing air;
2 noisy respiration with high-pitched sounds indicating the

31

most severe obstruction;

3 paradoxical breathing when inspiration results in the indrawing of the upper part of the chest and intercostal spaces;

4 tracheal tug in which the trachea is pulled down during inspiration due to uncoordinated respiratory muscle action.

The airway can be held open by pulling the jaw, and therefore the tongue which is attached to it, forwards. It is important to ensure that the correct body position is adopted to avoid aspiration of gastric contents, which will occur if the patient is left supine. The safest position is known as the 'coma' position, with the patient lying on the side with the head turned so that any pharyngeal contents will drain out of the mouth.

When brain stem reflex function is inadequate the lungs can be protected from aspiration of gastric contents most simply by intubation of the trachea with a cuffed endotracheal tube. The act of intubation itself, especially if a muscle relaxant drug is used, can result in massive aspiration unless cricoid pressure, which compresses the oesophagus, is applied by an assistant. In practice, the intubation of an unconscious patient with a potentially full stomach is hazardous. The patient should be pre-oxygenated for several minutes before intubation is attempted. As muscle paralysis is achieved prior to laryngoscopy, the oesophagus must be held closed to avoid aspiration of stomach contents. An assistant presses the cricoid cartilage firmly backwards as either consciousness is lost or, in the unconscious patient, the muscles become paralysed with a relaxant drug. The cricoid pressure should not be released until the endotracheal tube cuff is inflated.

If a cuffed tracheal tube is to be left for some time, it is better to select one of the plastic types which are less irritant to tissues, than the red rubber tubes commonly used during anaesthesia. After 10–14 days of nasotracheal intubation, a tracheostomy will usually need to be performed.

If the pressure in the cuff is too high there is a danger of tracheal mucosal ischaemia with sloughing, and eventual healing with fibrosis, causing tracheal stenosis. Latterly tubes have been produced with much longer and floppier cuffs, which need only be inflated with a low pressure and which adequately seal due to their large volume.

With endotracheal intubation, the patient is unable to cough due to the inability to seal the glottis, an essential part of the cough mechanism. Secretions accumulate in the respiratory passages and require to be sucked out regularly. Humidification of the inspired gases is important for longer-term ventilation.

When ventilation is controlled mechanically, the respiratory problems increase greatly. Respiratory parameters need to be monitored by regular measurements of arterial Po_2 and Pco_2 tensions.

THE HEART

The heart's function is continually monitored by ECG, blood pressure and pulse recordings. Adequacy of cardiac output can be indicated by a warm periphery. Body core/peripheral skin temperature gradient can be helpful to detect a falling cardiac output or hypovolaemia.

THE KIDNEYS

All unconscious patients need to be catheterized and the urine collected in a sterile container. Scrupulous attention to bladder sterility is vital. All urine passed is recorded.

FLUID BALANCE

Assuming normal renal function, fluid balance can be calculated fairly easily and any overhydration will be corrected by diuresis. A normal 70 kg person will require around 3 litres of water daily and will lose 1.5 litres as urine and 900 ml through the skin. Respiratory losses will depend on adequacy of humidification. Daily measurements of electrolytes, especially sodium, will indicate trends towards over or under hydration. Renal failure considerably complicates the management of the unconscious patient.

FEEDING

For long-term management, enteral feeding is obviously superior to parenteral. Although there are many proprietary enteral feeds available, larger hospitals employ dietitians whose advice should be sought, and who can arrange for appropriate tube feeding diets to be produced. Proprietary foods often seem to induce diarrhoea.

If alimentary function is diminished, parenteral feeding will be required. This should only be administered through a centrally placed venous cannula in either the subclavian or the external jugular vein to avoid peripheral venous thrombosis. The first principle is to provide sufficient calories, and then to add amino acids to diminish the negative nitrogen balance that usually occurs. Lipid feeds provide a rich source of energy. Long-term feeding regimes must recognize the importance of vitamins and contain trace elements.

NURSING

The success or failure of the management of the unconscious will ultimately depend on the skill and dedication of the nursing staff. Mouth toilet reduces the incidence of candida infections, and the eyes need to be kept closed to avoid drying of the cornea.

The skin is always at risk and if bedsores develop a patient becomes increasingly toxic. Bedsores usually develop in the skin overlying the sacrum and the buttocks or the heels. These areas need to be kept clean and dry. The use of air rings and ripple beds may help to maintain circulation through the skin in these dependent regions.

Pressure can cause damage to superficial nerves especially if they are overlying bone, such as the lateral popliteal nerve as it winds around the neck of the fibula — paralysis resulting in foot-drop.

If muscles and tendons are not stretched regularly by passive manipulation, fibrosis will occur resulting in permanent contractures and severe loss of function.

Chapter 7

Post-Operative Recovery

The post-operative recovery period after general anaesthesia is the transition between the time when the patient is fully anaesthetized, and the time when he is awake, pain-free, independent, mobile and taking a normal diet. At its simplest, this may be a matter of hours; after major abdominal or thoracic surgery it is usually days or sometimes weeks.

The recovery period may be divided into three phases: early, intermediate and late.

1 *In the early recovery period* the principle concern is usually the care of an unconscious patient, maintenance of the airway and ensuring that ventilation is adequate.

2 *In the intermediate recovery period* the patient is conscious and capable of maintaining his own airway. The problems are usually those of cardiovascular instability, the maintenance of renal function, ensuring that respiratory function is adequate and the establishment of effective analgesia.

3 *Late recovery* usually occurs on the surgical ward. Long-term fluid and electrolyte requirements have to be met, analgesia maintained, respiratory complications prevented, and a normal diet and normal mobility regained.

The early and intermediate recovery phases take place close to theatre, in a specifically designated recovery area staffed by experienced nurses with immediate access to medical (anaesthetic) assistance. Responsibility for a post-operative patient is formally handed over to the recovery staff by the anaesthetist, with instructions for management of the airway and respiration, fluid, electrolyte and blood administration and analgesia. The trolley or bed that the patient is nursed on must have the facility for a head-up and head-down tilt. There must be immediate access to:

1 high volume suction,
2 oxygen,
3 a means of delivering oxygen under positive pressure,

and the following must be close to hand:

1 equipment for endotracheal intubation, i.e. laryngoscope, endotracheal tubes, etc.,
2 intravenous fluids, administration sets and intravenous cannulae,
3 drugs and facilities for coping with a circulatory arrest — DC defibrillator, etc.,
4 a ventilator in case an extended period of ventilatory support is needed.

Management in the early and intermediate recovery phases is largely the concern of the anaesthetist, and will be discussed in terms of:

1 the respiratory system,
2 the cardiovascular system,
3 renal function,
4 fluid and electrolyte balance.

Post-operative analgesia will be discussed in Chapter 8.

THE RESPIRATORY SYSTEM

The airway

If unconscious, the patient is unable to maintain his airway and is at risk of respiratory obstruction, regurgitation and inhalation of stomach contents. If conscious, his level of consciousness is likely to be impaired and he is still at risk. Unless there are surgical contra-indications, all patients in the early recovery phase must be nursed on their side to prevent airway obstruction.

Ventilation

Ventilation (tidal volume and respiratory rate) must be adequate for gas exchange with enough reserve (vital capacity) to be able to cough adequately. If in doubt, these volumes can be measured with a simple flow meter, such as a Wright respirometer, attached to an anaesthetic mask. With a 70 kg adult, tidal volume should be at least 350 ml (5 ml/kg) and vital capacity 700 ml (10 ml/kg).

Common causes of ventilatory depression

At this time these are:
1 the effects of opiates administered intra-operatively,
2 residual neuromuscular blockade,
3 pain, and
4 hypocapnia after intra-operative hyperventilation.

Opiates such as morphine, pethidine, fentanyl etc., given for analgesia during surgery, may depress ventilation post-operatively. They can be reversed by naloxone but this also reverses the analgesia. Doxapram reverses respiratory depression without affecting analgesia but is only effective for a few minutes, so has to be given by continuous infusion.

Residual neuromuscular block is diagnosed by testing neuromuscular function with a peripheral nerve stimulator. Electrical stimulation of a motor nerve — e.g. the ulnar or the facial — results, in normal circumstances, in a vigorous contraction of the muscles it supplies. Neuromuscular blockade may be potentiated by electrolyte and acid base abnormalities and by large doses of some antibiotics.

Pain can inhibit ventilation. It is treated with analgesics, but analgesics themselves cause respiratory depression, so the dose has to be titrated against the desired response.

Hyperventilation, due to excessive intermittent positive pressure ventilation during surgery, can deplete the body's carbon dioxide stores and, until they are replenished, the patient may hypoventilate.

Post-operative oxygenation

Many patients have low arterial oxygen tensions for varying periods after their operation for a number of reasons:

Diffusion hypoxia occurs for up to 30 minutes after a period of nitrous oxide administration. Nitrous oxide which dissolves in body tissue during anaesthesia diffuses out into the alveoli and dilutes the alveolar gas. If the patient is breathing only room air, alveolar oxygen concentration will be undesirably low.

A decrease in lung volumes occurs after abdominal and thoracic surgery. After upper abdominal surgery vital capacity may decrease as much as 50–60%. This leads to a relative hypoventilation of alveoli at the base of the lung. It is usually manifest as a low arterial oxygen tension with a normal arterial carbon dioxide tension.

Respiratory depression due to the causes discussed earlier will cause primary hypoventilation. When this occurs hypoxaemia is accompanied by hypercarbia.

Healthy individuals usually tolerate the hypoxaemia after major surgery very well. Some patients however, are relatively hypoxaemic pre-operatively, such as the elderly — Pao_2 normally declines with age — and the pathologically obese. Patients with chronic chest disease are most often mildly hypoxaemic and normo- or hypocarbic. All these patients should be given oxygen routinely after surgery and in adequate amounts, i.e. 35–40%. The possibility of depressing the 'hypoxic drive' in patients with chest disease is relatively remote, although it does occur in a few individuals. These are usually patients who are severely hypoxaemic pre-operatively and have an elevated $Paco_2$. It should be possible to identify them pre-operatively. Hypoxaemia after major abdominal surgery is usually worst on the first and second post-operative days, then improves as lung volumes increase.

CARDIOVASCULAR SYSTEM

Hypotension after surgery is most commonly due to:
1 Hypovolaemia — blood lost during the course of surgery which has not been adequately replaced — and
2 anaesthetic and analgesic agents, which depress cardiac output and decrease the ability of the cardiovascular system to compensate for lesser degrees of hypovolaemia. Blood pressure usually recovers as the effects of the drugs wear off. Some anaesthetic agents stimulate the vagus and produce a bradycardia which can usually be effectively treated with atropine.

Persistent hypotension most often means inadequate fluid or blood replacement. If hypotension persists despite apparently adequate fluid replacement, other causes should be looked for, such as further concealed blood loss, myocardial infarction, heart failure or tension pneumothorax. A full 12-lead ECG should be performed and a chest X-ray taken. If seemingly large quantities of blood and fluid are infused with little apparent effect, central venous pressure should be monitored

RENAL FAILURE

Several factors in the peri-operative period reduce urine output. Blood loss, dehydration and hypotension cause a reduction in renal blood flow and in glomerular filtration rate. Part of the body's response to the surgical insult is an increase in the activity of aldosterone and antidiuretic hormone, resulting in fluid retention and diminished urine output. If left untreated, this may progress to acute tubular necrosis and established renal failure. A minimum urine flow of 25–30 ml/hour should be aimed for in the adult. Restoration of blood and fluid volume usually leads to restoration of urine output. If not, treatment with an osmotic or loop diuretic is indicated. If that does not succeed, treatment of acute renal failure will be instituted, possibly involving peritoneal or haemodialysis.

FLUIDS AND ELECTROLYTES

It is not the function of this book to discuss complex derangements of fluid and electrolyte and acid base balance. Provided all abnormal losses have been replaced pre-operatively and intra-operatively, and excluding continuing abnormal losses, the fluid and electrolyte requirements of a normal 70 kg adult unable to take anything by mouth are in the region of 2.5–3 litres of fluid a day, sodium 100–150 mmols/day, and potassium 60–80 mmols/day. These requirements are normally met by 2.5–3 litres of 0.18% saline in 4% dextrose solution over 24 hours, or 2 litres of 5% dextrose and 1 litre of 0.9% saline in 24 hours. Potassium administration is normally avoided in the first 24 hours after operation as there is usually a surfeit of circulating potassium ions from tissue damage incurred during the operation.

Chapter 8

Post-Operative Analgesia

Post-operative analgesia is required not only for humanitarian reasons but, particularly after thoracic and upper abdominal surgery, it allows the patient to breath adequately. It helps him cough and get rid of retained secretions, thereby avoiding chest complications.

Intramuscular opiates such as morphine and pethidine are the traditional way of giving post-operative analgesia. They should be administered regularly and before the pain returns. In practice, because of respiratory depression, this can be dangerous, unless the patient is closely supervised. The common practice is for opiates to be given as and when the patient asks. The problem is that delays usually occur, by which time the patient is often in some considerable distress. In these circumstances the analgesia is usually less effective.

Intravenous opiates can be given by continuous infusion using a pump but require close supervision because of the danger of respiratory depression.

On-demand intravenous analgesia has come into vogue recently. Metered doses of opiate are given by a syringe pump in response to the patient pressing a button to indicate he is in pain.

Epidural analgesia can be maintained post-operatively through an epidural cannula using either local analgesic agents or opiates. In the case of local analgesics, the cardiovascular system must be closely monitored because of the danger of hypotension. Epidural opiates have been introduced fairly recently. They have a prolonged duration of action and do not usually affect the cardiovascular system. However, they can produce severe respiratory depression which appears 8–12 hours after the opiate has been administered, possibly due to the drug tracking up to the brain stem. The chances of this occurring can be decreased by nursing the patient sitting upright.

Local nerve blocks can be used for pain relief following certain operations. One example is multiple intercostal nerve block after upper abdominal or thoracic surgery, although this can be complicated by pneumothorax. Other examples are ilio-inguinal block after inguinal hernia repair, or penile block after circumcision. Some surgeons may block the intercostal nerves under direct vision towards the end of a thoracic operation, and there has been a recent resurgence of interest in techniques of irrigating surgical wounds with local anaesthetic agents.

Chapter 9

Fluids, Electrolytes and Blood Transfusion

NORMAL FLUIDS AND ELECTROLYTE REQUIREMENTS

The normal fluid and electrolyte requirements of a fit 70 kg adult with a normal temperature and normal renal function are in the region of 2.5–3 litres of fluid, 100–150 mmols of sodium, and 60–80 mmols of potassium a day. If the patient is unable to take fluids by mouth but has no abnormal losses, these needs are usually met by 1 litre of 0.18% saline in 4% dextrose with 20 mmols of potassium chloride added to each litre and administered 8-hourly, or 2 litres of 5% dextrose and 1 litre of 0.9% saline in each 24 hours, again with 20 mmols of potassium chloride in each litre. The 5% dextrose is given not for its energy value, which is very small in relation to daily energy requirements, but for the water. The dextrose merely renders it iso-osmotic.

Usually patients having an elective operation have had nothing by mouth for at least 8 hours pre-operatively, and if their operation is late in the day, or has been delayed, then often for much longer. It can be expected they will arrive in theatre relatively dehydrated with a fluid deficit, in a normal size adult, of about 0.5–1 litre. If they have suffered abnormal losses, for example as a result of vomiting for 3 days or longer due to intestinal obstruction, they may be as much as 4–6 litres in deficit. Patients like this must be adequately rehydrated and resuscitated before operation.

During major surgery, in addition to appropriate replacement of blood loss, it is customary to administer balanced salt solution (Hartmanns or lactated Ringers) at a rate of about

5–15 ml/kg/hour. For a normal size otherwise healthy adult a simple regime would be 1 litre in the first hour and 500 ml/hour thereafter, depending on urine output. Balanced salt solution contains ions — potassium, calcium, chloride, etc. — in roughly the proportions present in plasma. Whether or not this has any definite advantage over 0.9% saline is still uncertain.

Because of the potential dangers and complications of blood transfusion, it is normal practice in a healthy individual not to replace blood during operation until up to 20% of the blood volume (in a normal size adult 1 litre) has been lost, and merely to replace the blood loss with clear fluid. Blood loss during surgery is estimated by weighing the swabs used and measuring the loss into the wound suction. This, however, does not take into account blood lost on the drapes and surgeons' gowns, and the figure obtained from weighing is usually considered to account for only 70–80% of the true loss.

Post-operatively, provided all losses have been replaced, fluid requirements are met by the 2.5–3 litre a day regimen discussed earlier, plus an allowance for continuing abnormal losses, such as nasogastic suction or fistula loss.

BLOOD TRANSFUSION

There is no doubt that replacement with whole blood is still the best treatment of severe acute blood loss. Previously healthy individuals, with a normal haemoglobin, can lose up to 20% of their circulating blood volume and have it replaced with non-oxygen-carrying alternatives — clear fluids, dextrans, starch gels, etc. When blood loss is greater than that or patients have haemoglobin concentrations lower than the normal range, blood lost should be replaced with whole blood.

Blood for transfusion is taken from the donor into preservative which includes an anticoagulant, an energy source and a buffer and is stored at 4°C. Blood is a living tissue. During its storage it is still metabolically active and, as it ages, it deteriorates. Formed elements disintegrate, energy substrates are used up, hydrogen ions accumulate and intracellular potassium becomes extracellular. The pH of 3-week-old blood is about 6.6 and the potassium concentration in the plasma in the region of 30 mmol/l. Blood is taken from the fridge at 4°C and should be warmed to 37°C immediately before infusion, usually by passing through a blood-warming coil immersed in a water bath.

Complications of blood transfusion

One of the most serious potential complications of blood transfusion is mismatch due to clerical error or failure to check the blood adequately against the patient's details before administration, resulting in the wrong unit of blood being given to the patient. Apart from this catastrophe the other complications of blood transfusion include:

1 Infection or transmission of disease either from the donor, e.g. viral hepatitis, syphilis, malaria, acquired immunodeficiency syndrome etc., or due to contamination in the taking or storage.

2 Incompatibility or haemolytic reactions leading to release of free haemoglobin and subsequent renal failure.

3 Allergic reactions — often mild urticarial reactions are of little clinical significance and controlled with antihistamines.

4 Citrate toxicity, potassium intoxication and acidity. Citrate potassium and hydrogen ions are all present in high concentration in stored blood. The citrate and potassium are myocardial depressants, and it is common practice that with large rapid transfusions 1g of calcium gluconate should be given with every litre of blood transfused. When citrate is metabolized hydrogen ions are eliminated, and it is common for a metabolic alkalosis to be present the day after a large blood transfusion.

5 Microaggregate debris — in stored blood, aggregates of fibrin, platelets and red cells form over a period. If these are transfused directly into the venous system they pass to the pulmonary circulation where they get trapped and may cause damage. These aggregates have been implicated in the aetiology of 'shock lung' (see Chapter 10). When any transfusion is given, it is now customary to pass the blood through a fine screen filter with pores of 20 or 40μm before administering it to the patient.

Chapter 10

Intercurrent Disease Affecting Anaesthesia and Surgery

Many patients presenting for elective surgery suffer from chronic medical illnesses and are receiving drug treatment. The problems of cardiovascular and respiratory disease were discussed in Chapter 5. This chapter deals with the problems associated with a number of diseases of other systems. For any patient with a medical condition who needs an operation, the dangers of operating should be set against the prognosis or the quality of life if the operation is not carried out, and given the situation, the patient should be in the best condition possible. To this end the advice and co-operation of a physician — preferably the physician who normally looks after that patient — should be sought to determine, given the time and the facilities available, whether the patient's condition could still be improved prior to the operation. The pros and cons of operating or not operating must also be discussed with the patient and/or if necessary his relatives. It is, after all, the patient's life that is at risk and the ultimate decision must rest with him or her.

ENDOCRINE DISORDERS

Diabetes mellitus

Diabetes is potentially one of the most serious of the medical conditions encountered in patients undergoing surgery. The acute dangers are:
1 unrecognized hypoglycaemia during the operation;
2 destabilization of the diabetes caused by the surgery and reduced or absent oral intake post-operatively.
   The more long-term dangers are those of the complications of diabetes — renal disease, hypertension, heart failure. Surgery

and trauma produce insulin resistance for reasons which are not entirely clear, and insulin requirements during and after operation increase. Keto acidosis takes several hours to develop, so with elective surgery it is usually some time after the patient has returned to the ward that problems arise. If the patient has been acutely ill before operation, then unless the insulin dosage has already been adjusted the problem of keto acidosis may already exist. However, the problem of unrecognized hypoglycaemia occurring intra-operatively is usually of more immediate concern to the anaesthetist. Over recent years, with the development of bedside methods of monitoring blood sugar such as Dextrostix and the use of glucose and insulin infusions given by a reliable electrical or mechanical pump to control blood sugar, this has ceased to be a major problem.

With diabetics maintained on diet and oral hypoglycaemic agents, both breakfast and the hypoglycaemic agent are commonly omitted the morning of operation. Blood sugar is monitored during the operation and urinary ketones if the surgery is major and prolonged. There are rarely any problems. If hypoglycaemia or keto acidosis develops, they can be dealt with in the conventional fashion.

With diabetics on soluble insulin, it was a common practice to administer a reduced dose of insulin the morning of operation, and to start an intravenous infusion of 5% dextrose at the same time. It is now more usual to omit the morning insulin dose and to start an infusion of 10–20% dextrose containing insulin and potassium, or to administer insulin concurrently from a syringe pump. The quantity of insulin given in relation to the glucose will depend on the severity of the diabetes. Blood sugar is monitored throughout and the insulin infusion rate adjusted accordingly. The glucose and insulin infusion is continued until the patient's oral intake has returned to normal. Alternatively, frequent (3-hourly) low insulin doses can be given subcutaneously or intramuscularly over the post-operative period, depending on the blood sugar, urinary sugar and urinary ketone levels— the so-called sliding scale.

Adrenocortical insufficiency and steroid replacement therapy

Many patients are taking cortisol or related drugs for a wide variety of reasons — rheumatoid arthritis, asthma, ulcerative colitis, leukaemia, organ transplantation, etc. Chronic cortisol therapy produces depression of the adrenal cortex so that the normal adrenocortical response to the stress of surgery is impaired. For many years it has been customary to increase steroid administration to cover the operation and the postoperative period. When the patient is able to take the drug by mouth, extra steroid cover is provided by increasing his normal dosage. Hydrocortisone 100 mg intramuscularly with the premedication, and 6-hourly thereafter either intramuscularly or in the intravenous infusion, is a common regimen to cover the peri-operative period until the patient is able to take something by mouth. It is uncertain how necessary this is for patients who have taken steroids in the past but are no longer doing so. Certainly most anaesthetists would agree that a regimen of this type should be followed by anyone taking steroids at the time of the operation, and probably anyone who had been taking them up to 6 months previously. Beyond that, the necessity is uncertain. The principal sign of adrenal insufficiency in these circumstances is persistent and otherwise unexplained hypotension.

Thyroid disease

Myxoedematous and hyperthyroid patients should be euthyroid before operation. Thyrotoxicosis is associated with high levels of sympathetic activity — tachycardia, sweating, etc. — and there is a danger of tachyarrhythmias and ventricular fibrillation. If on treatment, they may be taking beta-blockers which also present problems. A bulky thyroid, particularly if it extends retrosternally, may compress the trachea and cause obstruction, so all such patients should have their neck and thoracic inlet X-rayed pre-operatively.

RENAL DISEASE AND RENAL FUNCTION

A number of factors during anaesthesia and surgery affect renal function and depress urine output. Both renal blood flow

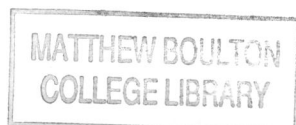

and glomerular filtration rate decrease. Surgery promotes secretion of antidiuretic hormone and aldosterone promoting the
reabsorption of sodium and water. If urine flow is not maintained, temporary cessation of urine output due to the above
factors — so called pre-renal renal failure — may progress to
established renal failure. Urine output should be maintained
by ensuring adequate hydration, avoiding hypotension and, if
necessary, by the judicious use of a diuretic. Patients at risk
from renal failure in the peri-operative period are those with
already impaired renal function, patients undergoing aortic
surgery, particularly where the renal blood supply is inter-
rupted, those having operations on the urinary tract, patients
who have suffered a period of haemorrhaghic shock, and jaundiced patients. This latter group are particularly at risk for
reasons that are still not certain, but with jaundiced patients
active steps should be taken to maintain urine flow by infusion
of fluids (and by an osmotic diuretic such as mannitol) started
pre-operatively and continued well into the post-operative
period.

Chronic renal failure and anephric patients

With the widespread use of haemodialysis, patients on dialysis
may need to be anaesthetized. The problems of anaesthetizing
dialysis patients are greatest with those who have not been
dialysed for several days — fluid overload, hypertension and
pulmonary oedema. Many patients with chronic renal disease
are taking antihypertensive drugs, most frequently beta-
blockers, as well as other drugs such as steroids and other
immunosuppressants. They are unable to excrete drugs
efficiently so dosages are reduced. Patients with a successful
transplant can be treated as normal.

LIVER DISEASE

Many patients with liver disease have abnormalities of their
blood clotting mechanisms because of poor vitamin K absorption from the gut due to a shortage of bile salts. Vitamin K
should be given by injection pre-operatively. Drug metabolism
may be impaired in patients with poor hepatic function, so the
action of analgesics may persist for an inordinate length of

time. Anaesthesia and surgery produce disturbances in portal venous and hepatic blood flow so surgery may be followed by a deterioration in liver function.

OBESITY

Obesity presents many problems for both the anaesthetist and the surgeon, and is associated with a higher morbidity and mortality. Obese patients who are to have elective surgery should lose as much weight as possible before operation. There are technical problems in operating through layers of fat several inches thick, and the incidence of wound infections and wound dehiscence is greater, as is the incidence of chest complications, deep vein thrombosis and pulmonary embolus.

For the anaesthetist the technical problems include finding veins and maintaining the airway. Obesity produces a restrictive defect in pulmonary mechanics so the work of breathing is increased. Lung volumes — total lung capacity, vital capacity and functional residual capacity — are decreased and the obese patient is relatively hypoxaemic. Arterial carbon dioxide tensions are generally normal or may be low. Because of the increased respiratory load, most anaesthetists would choose to ventilate morbidly obese patients even for short operations. Rarely the chronic hypoxaemia may be associated with pulmonary hypertension and congestive cardiac failure, peripheral oedema and the somnolence of the Pickwickian (obesity hypoventilation) syndrome. In this instance the hypoxaemia is more severe than in simple obesity and is associated 'with carbon dioxide retention.

Obese individuals can be operated on satisfactorily under local anaesthesia, using epidural or spinal for abdominal surgery, but there are obvious technical difficulties in identifying landmarks to determine the correct site for the local anaesthetic injection. If a local block can be established and maintained for some time after abdominal or thoracic surgery this is of obvious benefit because of the diminished respiratory function associated with this type of operation.

Post-operatively, obese patients should be given supplementary oxygen and nursed sat upright to optimize arterial oxygenation. If the obesity hypoventilation syndrome is present supplementary oxygen would probably depress ventilation, but difficulty may also be experienced in restoring spontaneous ventilation in patients with this syndrome after a prolonged period of IPPV. Patients with the obesity hypoventilation syndrome present a very serious problem for major surgery.

CENTRAL NERVOUS SYSTEM DISORDERS

Epilepsy

Most anaesthetic drugs depress the cerebral cortex and have a beneficial effect upon seizure disorders. However, some — ethrane, methohexitone, etomidate and althesin — also have excitatory effects, can exacerbate epileptic states and should be avoided. Blood gas abnormalities — hypoxia, hyper or hypocarbia — can have the same effect. Care should also be exercised when using local anaesthetic agents because of their propensity to cause convulsions. The patient's anti-epileptic drugs must be continued over the period of the operation and given parenterally when he or she is unable to take them orally.

Chronic neurological disorders

Chronic neurological disorders such as multiple sclerosis or motor neurone disease are sometimes exacerbated by anaesthesia and surgery.

Cerebrovascular disease

Patients with cerebrovascular insufficiency may show a deterioration in their condition after operation especially if wide variations in blood pressure have been allowed to occur.

MUSCLE DISORDERS

The various muscle disorders such as the muscular dystrophies, Pompes disease, dystrophia myotonica, and the malignant hyperpyrexia myopathy, etc. all present very serious problems in relation to surgery and anaesthesia. Many myopathies affect the myocardium in addition to skeletal muscle. The principle complications are respiratory failure due to muscle weakness, as well as heart failure and cardiac arrest, and these can occur many hours after the operation.

OLD AGE

As anaesthetic and surgical techniques have improved, more and more elderly people are now having quite major surgery, particularly procedures such as total hip replacement. The elderly have a general slowing down of all bodily functions in addition to a higher incidence of intercurrent disease, although surprisingly little is known about the normal physiology of old age. Cardiac output is decreased and the circulation time slower, exercise tolerance is diminished, and body fat (the body's energy store) is decreased so they tolerate periods of starvation less readily. Metabolic rate is slower and thermoregulatory mechanisms are impaired. Arterial oxygen tension declines with age, so with the decrease in arterial Po_2 after major abdominal surgery they can be quite severely hypoxaemic. Generally speaking, their ability to cope with the insults of injury or surgery is diminished. They are often more sensitive to anaesthetic and sedative drugs, and metabolize them more slowly than a younger person. They may also become disorientated and confused by the unfamiliar environment.

Chapter 11

Complications of Anaesthesia

Complications are seen in all branches of practical medicine resulting from mistakes, unpredictable happenings, idiosyncrasies, hypersensitivities and, regrettably, negligence. Every manoeuvre, every drug, every event carries with it the risk of potential complications. In this chapter some of the commoner ones which the medical student is likely to see will be mentioned together with the causes!

PHYSICAL DAMAGE

Blood vessels

Faulty technique in venepuncture can result in bruising, extravasation of drugs which can cause ulceration of the overlying skin, localized infection, thrombophlebitis and damage to adjacent structures, especially arteries and nerves. Injections and drugs should be into superficial veins which can easily be palpated, and as remote as possible from arteries such as the brachial artery. Some drugs, including the benzodiazepines and propanidid, cause thrombophlebitis. Prolonged venous cannulation is more likely to result in thrombophlebitis and infection. Especially important is the risk of septicaemia from septic emboli from the end of the venous cannula.

Central venous cannulation is comparatively hazardous causing perforation of large intrathoracic or cervical veins and pneumothorax.

Arterial puncture, and especially cannulation, is associated with arterial thrombosis and thromboembolic phenomena producing painful Osler's nodes in the fingers.

Intubation

Trivial but unnecessary damage to lips and gums is a frequent accompaniment of inexperienced intubation of the trachea. More serious is damage to the teeth with the potential for inhalation of the detached fragments followed by lung abscess if left undetected. Nasotracheal intubation can cause an inconvenient epistaxis, and on occasions the tube can tunnel its way under the nasal mucosa; nasal intubation often fractures the turbinates. Damage to tonsils and laryngeal structures especially the vocal cords is fortunately rare, but rough handling of posterior oral structures contributes to sore throat post-operatively.

Superficial nerves

Direct sustained pressure will damage nerves, such as: the lateral popliteal as it winds round the head of the fibula, causing foot drop; the facial as it crosses the mandible, causing facial muscle paralysis; the ulnar as it crosses the medial epichondyle, causing paralysis of and loss of sensation in the hand; and the radial nerve as it winds round the humerus posteriorly, causing wrist drop. The brachial plexus can be damaged by stretching it over the head of the humerus if the arm is too far abducted or externally rotated.

The eyes

In the unconscious patient the eyes are usually kept closed by applying either tape or eye pads to avoid corneal drying and corneal abrasion, which can easily happen if the head is covered by drapes.

Electrical

The risk of electrocution is always present, especially when more than one electronic device is attached to a patient. The usual cause is faulty earthing, although comparatively small electric currents across the heart can cause ventricular fibrillation. Faults in the earth plate or lead to the diathermy machine result in other return pathways for the diathermy current and this, if a small skin area is involved, will cause burns which can penetrate to include deep structures such as blood vessels.

RESPIRATORY

The complication most feared by undergraduates and trainee anaesthetists is acute respiratory obstruction during or shortly after induction of anaesthesia. Laryngeal spasm and breath holding can be difficult to differentiate, and can occur as a response to light anaesthesia, especially if the airway is stimulated by irritant anaesthetic vapours or foreign material including secretions and acid gastric contents. Failed intubation can become a nightmare when gastric aspiration is likely, as with unprepared emergencies and obstetric patients. The latter group are very prone to develop Mendelson's syndrome, characterized by bronchospasm, cyanosis and cardiovascular collapse — as discussed more fully elsewhere.

Respiratory failure is largely a post-operative phenomenon due usually to a combination of events. Muscle weakness after inadequate reversal of relaxants, central depression with both opioids and anaesthetics, inhibition of coughing and inadequate alveolar ventilation secondary to wound pain combine to produce a restrictive respiratory failure with CO_2 retention and eventually CO_2 narcosis, especially if the P_{O_2} is maintained with oxygen administration.

Sudden respiratory embarrassment, especially ocurring later in convalescence, is usually as a result of pulmonary embolism secondary to the detachment of a thrombus from either the calf or a pelvic vein. Deep vein thrombosis in the legs can be suspected when the patient complains of swelling or tenderness of the calf muscles; Homan's sign is usually positive. Pulmonary embolism may present as a haemoptysis or as a generalized collapse similar to a major myocardial infarction, from which it is sometimes hard to differentiate.

CARDIOVASCULAR

Hypotension during surgery is not infrequent particularly in the elderly and the very ill. Sudden blood loss during vascular surgery is especially liable to render the cardiovascular system unstable. Undesirable results of severe and prolonged hypotension are brain damage with or without venous thrombosis, and renal impairment. The former may result in a delayed return of consciousness, and the latter will not be fully appreciated until some hours after surgery.

Contrary to popular lay belief, the heart is an extremely robust organ which can withstand severe short-lived insults such as hypotension and hypoxia. Nevertheless, when the coronary circulation is compromised with atheroma, the incidence of myocardial infarction is greatly increased. A previous myocardial infarction within the last 6 months is associated with a greatly increased incidence of further post-operative infarction. Surgery should be delayed if possible for over a year when the dangers are little greater than normal. Myocardial infarction may well occur as a response to stress and so local anaesthesia is unlikely to protect the patient — contrary to the view of some surgeons who assume that the general anaesthetic is the cause. Hypotension in the sitting subject whether anaesthetized (e.g. dental patients) or conscious (e.g. post-operatively) may result in severe cerebral ischaemia and fainting.

HEPATIC

The cause of post-operative hepatitis has been furiously debated for over a quarter of a century since the introduction of halothane. It is likely that halothane can cause hepatitis but is very uncommon. The incidence of the active hepatitis A virus in the general population is probably much commoner, being estimated to be around 100–400 per million at any one time. It may be that anaesthetics reduce the efficacy of the immune system and render a patient more liable to infections including viral hepatitis. Repeat halothane anaesthetics within a 6-week interval should perhaps be discouraged.

BODY TEMPERATURE

Anaesthesia, by virtue of the invariable peripheral venodilatation it produces, results in a fall of body core temperature. During prolonged surgery, especially with exposure of viscera, severe hypothermia may develop, resulting in delayed return of consciousness, inadequate respiration and peripheral perfusion. The respiratory problems will be compounded if oxygen demand is increased as a consequence of shivering during the post-operative period. High body temperature may occur with a blood transfusion reaction to certain drugs. The most serious form of raised body temperature is called malignant hyperpyrexia (MH), which is often fatal and affects young fit adults who have inherited the susceptibility. In MH the body temperature may reach non-viable levels of 45°C within 1–2 hours of the commencement of anaesthesia. Patients also develop severe acidosis, hyperkalaemia, muscle spasm and myoglobinuria which can cause obstructive renal failure. The disease is treated effectively with intravenous dantrolene if the diagnosis is made before irreversible changes have occurred.

Chapter 12

Local Anaesthesia

Local anaesthetics are used in all branches of medical practice to produce nerve blockade, and in cardiology to control arrhythmias; in some centres they are used as systemic analgesics.

CHEMISTRY

Most local anaesthetics consist of three parts:

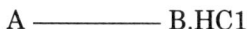

$$A \text{———} B.HCl$$

Radical A is lipophilic and is attracted to lipid structures such as cell membranes. Radical B is hydrophilic and forms electrostatic bonds in acid solution to produce a salt. The chemical chain between the two radicals usually contains either an esteratic link as in procaine and amethocaine (Tetracaine), or an amide link as in lignocaine (Xylocaine), prilocaine (Citanest), bupivacaine (Marcaine) and cinchocaine (Nupercaine).

MECHANISM OF ACTION

Nearly all the common local anaesthetics are weak bases which form acid salts. After injection they dissociate liberating a base which, as it is uncharged, can diffuse across membranes. The uncharged base accepts a hydrogen ion and as an acid cation is pharmacologically active. It is now accepted that local anaesthetics exert their pharmacological effects on the inside of the cell membranes by reducing ionic conductance and permeability and thus causing stabilization of the membrane potential. If the cell concerned is a nerve cell or its axon, it will

57

lose its ability to generate and to conduct nerve impulses. The degree of dissociation depends on the pH of the extracellular fluid, and in acidic tissue such as in the vicinity of infected tissue, local anaesthetics may be much less effective.

LATENCY

After administration, the time of onset of a nerve block depends inversely on the concentration of the solution, on the pH of the tissue and on the diameter of the nerve fibres; smaller nerves are blocked before larger nerves. It is possible to block differentially the smaller pain fibres (A delta and C fibres) whilst leaving the larger motor and proprioceptive fibres unaffected. The latency, in practice, depends largely on the distance the local anaesthetic drug solution has to diffuse to reach the nerve fibres.

DURATION

Duration of action depends firstly on the affinity of the lipophilic radical to the lipoproteins in the cell membrane, secondly on the loss of drug, by diffusion, into the local blood circulation, and thirdly on the concentration of local anaesthetic drug used.

Adrenaline is often added to local anaesthetic drug solutions to reduce local blood flow and thereby to prolong the action. Cocaine differs from other local anaesthetics as it has vasoconstrictor properties; all the others cause vasodilation.

METABOLISM AND EXCRETION

The drugs with an esteratic linkage are broken down by plasma esterases; competition for esterases by anticholinesterases and other ester drugs, such as propanidid, can prolong the action of these local anaesthetics. The amide linkage drugs are broken down in the microsomes in the liver, and sometimes also in the kidneys. Procaine and amethocaine should not be used when a patient is receiving a sulphonamide.

If a vasoconstrictor is added the doses shown in Table 12.1 can be exceeded. The usual vasoconstrictor is adrenaline 1:200,000 final concentration. The maximum dose of adrenaline is 0.5 mg for the average adult. 20 ml of 1% lignocaine solution contains 200 mg.

Table 12.1. Local anaesthetic dosages

Drug	Maximum dose (mg/kg)	Solution strength (%)	
		Injection	Surface
Cocaine	3	NA	10
Procaine	10	0.5–2	—
Amethocaine	4	0.05–0.1	0.05
Lignocaine	3	0.5–2	4
Prilocaine	6	1.5–3	—
Bupivacaine	2	0.1	0.1
Cinchocaine	1	0.05–0.1	0.1

TOXICITY

1 *CNS.* Stimulation with muscle fasiculations and restlessness leading to convulsions. Depression with unconsciousness and respiratory failure.

2 *CVS.* Hypotension, bradycardia, pallor and sweating leading to cardiorespiratory arrest.

3 *Allergy.* Anaphylactoid reaction with bronchospasm, angioneurotic oedema and hypotension.

4 *Vasoconstrictor.* Adrenaline causes hypertension, tachycardia and anxiety when given intravenously.

All toxic reactions are more marked in the old and debilitated, and especially if the injection is given intravenously by mistake, or into a very vascular part of the body where absorption is rapid. Adrenaline should never be used in fingers, toes and penis due to the risk of end-artery spasm and gangrene.

USES OF LOCAL ANAESTHETICS

Field blocks

Surface anaesthesia is mainly restricted to membranes within the orifices, and the cornea. Cocaine 10% is very effective but is more toxic than the others. If cocaine is to be used a 10 mg i.m. test dose is given and a rise in heart rate of 15 b.p.m. indicates hypersensitivity.

Infiltration anaesthesia is very effective, but often requires a large volume if the surgical area is extensive and may hinder surgery due to tissue bogginess, and it delays healing.

Intravenous local anaesthesia (Bier's block) is used in a limb rendered ischaemic with a tourniquet. It is very useful for surgery of the hand and forearm. If the tourniquet is released too early, systemic toxicity occurs and deaths have been reported. Though technically easy, the dangers are such that the block should only be performed by an experienced anaesthetist.

Nerve blocks

A nerve block is used to produce anaesthesia in the distribution of that nerve and is known as a field block. Nerve blocks often have to be multiple, such as a wrist block which involves ulnar, median and radial nerves. Specific nerve blocks are difficult and demand a good knowledge of anatomy. The easiest nerves to block individually are the intercostals. One major advantage over infiltration blocks is that less local anaesthetic drug is used.

Plexus blocks are frequently used, especially the brachial plexus for upper arm limb surgery. The supraclavicular approach may result in pneumothorax and phrenic nerve palsy and should never be performed bilaterally. The axillary approach may result in patchy anaesthesia if the musculocutaneous nerve takes off at a higher level than the blocked region. A coracoid approach has recently been described which avoids these complications as does the scalene approach commonly used in the USA.

Spinal anaesthesia

Subarachnoid spinal block

This is achieved when a local anaesthetic drug is injected into the CSF using a lumbar puncture technique; anaesthesia develops rapidly. This route has been used in man since 1898 (Bier) though has never achieved great popularity in the UK, where general anaesthesia has been preferred. The only type of subarachnoid spinal likely to be seen nowadays is for lower abdominal, genital, anal and leg surgery. The extent of the block depends on:
1   dose of drug used;

2 volume of anaesthetic solution;
3 babotage — mixing of drug with CSF during injection;
4 position of patient during and after injection;
5 density of drug solution — hyperbaric solutions fall.

The duration of the block depends also on the drug chosen. Heavy nupercaine is commonly used though lignocaine and bupivacaine preparations are also becoming popular.

Immediate complications are generally related to sympathetic blockade which often occurs at a higher level than indicated by dermatome anaesthesia, as the sympathetic preganglionic nerves have small diameters and are blocked by a drug concentration too low to cause somatic nerve blockade. Severe hypotension will require head-down tilt, i.v. fluids and a vasopressor.

Later complications include headache due to CSF leakage at the puncture site, backache due to local damage, sphincter disturbances, abducent nerve palsy causing squint (this is probably due to this long intracranial nerve being stretched over the wing of the sphenoid when an excessive volume of CSF is lost), and rarely meningitis.

Epidural anaesthesia

This can be produced at any level although the commonest sites are lumbar and caudal. Although local anaesthetic drugs have been injected into the epidural space in man since 1921 (Pages), this route has only achieved great popularity over the last two decades, probably as a result of the greater availability of longer lasting drugs. Epidural anaesthesia has been found to be especially valuable in obstetrics both for normal vaginal delivery and latterly for caesarian section.

The lumbar epidural space is usually identified using a blunt needle (Tuohy) which will not pierce the dura, and a catheter is left in situ so that further 'top-ups' can be made either for prolonged surgery or post-operative analgesia. The local anaesthetic solution gains access to the segmental nerves as they cross from the intrathecal space to the intervertebral foramina. The somatic level of anaesthesia depends mainly on the volume injected, and the duration of block on the drug used. Adrenaline can be added to increase the duration of block, although this is not necessary if a catheter has been placed.

The caudal epidural space is approached through the sacro-coccygeal membrane which covers the sacral hiatus. Occasionally caudal blocks are unsatisfactory and anaesthesia is patchy due to fibrous tissue membranes within the caudal canal. The complications include sympathetic blockade causing hypotension (especially if the drug is allowed to block the lower thoracic spinal nerves), dural tap (with similar problems as in intrathecal blocks), total spinal blockade by injecting by mistake into the subarachnoid space, and backache due to direct trauma to ligaments and muscle tissues.

Autonomic blockade

Sympathetic ganglion blocks are used therapeutically to control pain and to induce vasodilation to increase blood flow. The stellate ganglion is easily blocked as it lies anterior to the 7th cervical and 1st thoracic transverse processes, which can be palpated. The lumbar sympathetic chain is blocked by a paravertebral approach to L2, 3, and 4 vertebrae and the coeliac plexus lies anterior to the aorta at the level of T12 and L1.

Chapter 13

Cardiovascular Monitoring

The lowest common denominator of cardiovascular function is cardiac output and it is to the maintenance of cardiac output and to the perfusion of vascular beds most sensitive to hypoxia that most aspects of cardiovascular function are directed. Cardiac output is measured using the Fick principle or by dye dilution. Neither of them are in routine clinical use as a monitoring technique although 'thermal dilution', a variation on the dye dilution method, is being used more and more frequently on intensive care and during major surgery of patients with heart disease. The technique is discussed later in this chapter.

During major surgery the following cardiovascular parameters are routinely monitored and to a greater or lesser degree bear some relationship to cardiac output and peripheral tissue perfusion:

1 blood pressure;
2 heart rate;
3 ECG;
4 central venous pressure;
5 urine output;
6 central–peripheral temperature gradients.

BLOOD PRESSURE

This is related to cardiac output by way of peripheral resistance. Cardiac output can drop precipitously but provided a compensatory rise in peripheral resistance occurs there may be little or no change in blood pressure. Likewise, if peripheral resistance falls and cardiac output remains the same blood pressure may fall quite markedly.

63

Blood pressure is normally measured indirectly using a sphygmomanometer. For critically ill patients on intensive care, for operations involving an inevitable heavy blood loss such as arterial surgery or for an operation where a patient's blood pressure may change markedly from second to second, either intentionally, such as during controlled hypotension for intracranial aneurysm surgery, or because of their condition (cardiac surgery), it is now usual practice to monitor arterial pressure directly using a cannula placed in a suitable artery. The radial or brachial arteries are normally used, although the dorsalis pedis is equally acceptable. The cannula is connected to a pressure transducer by a length of tubing kept filled and continuously flushed with heparinized saline. The transducer changes the mechanical energy of the arterial pressure wave to an electrical signal displayed on an oscilloscope or converted to a digital display of systolic, diastolic or mean arterial blood pressure. Intra-arterial monitoring is expensive in terms of the capital equipment required and has a morbidity in terms of thrombosis of the artery. The chances of thrombosis are greater the longer the arterial cannula is in place, the larger it is and the smaller the artery into which it is inserted.Thrombosis may be followed by necrotic changes in tissues that the artery supplies. For this reason it is most commonly placed in the radial artery, as the hand usually has a collateral arterial supply via the ulnar artery. The brachial and femoral arteries are both end arteries, so although they are less likely to thrombose because of their size, if they did so the consequences would be disastrous.

HEART RATE

This is directly related to cardiac output by way of stroke volume. By increasing in the face of a decrease in stroke volume, due say to haemorrhage, cardiac output can be maintained.

ECG

The ECG is an indication of the electrical activity in the heart and normally bears no direct relationship to cardiac output, although the presence of ventricular fibrillation or asystole obviously denotes an absence of output. It is monitored to detect arrythmias and ischaemic changes in the myocardium.

CENTRAL VENOUS PRESSURE

The central venous pressure (CVP) is the pressure in the great veins filling the right atrium, i.e. the superior or inferior vena cava, but corresponds also to right atrial diastolic pressure. It is a measure of the filling pressure of the right side of the heart and is an index of venous return. In terms of the Starling relationship cardiac output is directly related to venous return. CVP is therefore affected by all the factors that affect venous return and cardiac filling, such as blood volume, venous tone, position, intrathoracic pressure and myocardial contractility. Central venous pressure is normally measured using a saline manometer attached to a cannula passed into the superior vena cava, either using a long line from the antecubital fossa or a shorter cannula inserted via the subclavian vein or the internal jugular. It can also be passed via the femoral vein into the inferior vena cava, but this site is more prone to infection and is not commonly used.

URINE PRODUCTION

With a normal kidney urine flow is the ultimate index of cardiovascular function and tissue perfusion. If the patient is catheterized and urine output being monitored, a minimum flow of 0.5 ml/kg/hour should be aimed for, or at least 25–30 ml/hour in the normal sized adult. No urine passed at all usually means the catheter is blocked, but a flow rate lower than 25–30 ml/hour should be treated by firstly ensuring adequate rehydration, then possibly stimulating renal function with an osmotic diuretic such as mannitol or a loop diuretic such as frusemide.

CENTRAL–PERIPHERAL TEMPERATURE GRADIENTS

The gradient between central temperature, as measured in the rectum, the nasophyaynx, the oesophagus, or the ear, and the temperature measured at a peripheral site such as the big toe, or the thumb, in a normovolaemic person, in a thermoneutral environment is normally about 2–3°C. Factors which increase this gradient are those which produce peripheral vasoconstriction by stimulating the sympathetic nervous system, namely hypovolaemia, cold, pain, fear and anxiety. The temperature gradient is therefore a useful index of how well peripheral tissues are being perfused, and changes in the gradient indicate corresponding changes in peripheral perfusion.

PULMONARY CAPILLARY WEDGE PRESSURE

This is a measurement now coming into routine use in critically ill patients on intensive care, in cardiac surgery and in patients with severe heart disease undergoing major surgery. The pulmonary capillary wedge pressure very closely reflects left atrial filling pressure, which is an index of venous return to the left side of the heart, in the same way as central venous pressure is an index of venous return to the right side of the heart. Its measurement relies on the fact that the pulmonary circulation is a low pressure circulation, so that if a branch of the pulmonary artery is occluded, the pressure in the artery distal to the occlusion reflects the pressure in the pulmonary veins which enter the left atrium on the other side of the pulmonary capillary bed. It is useful when administering fluids to patients with impaired left ventricular function, and allows fluid to be administered up to the point at which left atrial filling pressure increases beyond the point at which back pressure on the pulmonary capillary bed would produce pulmonary oedema.

In practice, pulmonary capillary wedge pressure is measured by passing a Swan-Ganz catheter through the right side of the heart into the pulmonary artery. This is a catheter with a small inflatable balloon on the tip. The balloon is inflated and 'wedged' in a small branch of the pulmonary artery. The lumen of the catheter opens distal to the balloon and the pressure distal to the balloon can be measured through the lumen. With the balloon blocking off a branch of the pulmonary artery, this pressure is a measure of the pressure in the pulmonary capillary bed as described above.

CARDIAC OUTPUT

Using a modified Swan-Ganz catheter in the pulmonary artery, cardiac output can be measured using thermal dilution. The technque is a variation on the classical dye dilution method of measuring cardiac output. A known quantity of ice cold saline is injected as a bolus through the catheter. This bolus leaves the catheter at an exit port partway along its length and the change in temperature produced by the saline is measured by a thermistor at the catheter tip. The electrical signal from the thermistor is fed directly into a computer or dedicated microprocessor. From a knowledge of exactly how much saline was injected and from the pattern of temperature change measured by the thermistor with respect to time (the area under the curve), the microprocessor calculates cardiac output.

Chapter 14

'Shock'

Shock can be defined as a failure of oxygenation of the peripheral tissues due to a failure in peripheral perfusion. In clinical practice the term is normally used to denote acute arterial hypotension accompanied by pallor, cold clammy peripheries and a rapid thready pulse. It may be due to a number of causes and is commonly classified by its aetiology.

AETIOLOGY

Haemorrhagic or hypovolaemic shock

This is due to acute loss of blood or tissue fluids. This type of shock has been the most thoroughly investigated and many of its features are common to the other types. With acute blood loss, blood pressure is maintained by an increase in activity of the sympathetic nervous system. Peripheral vasoconstriction occurs, shunting blood from relatively non-essential tissues such as the skin and gut, and preserving the perfusion of those tissues most sensitive to hypoxia such as the brain, the heart and the kidneys. Hydrostatic pressure in the capillaries drops and fluid from the interstitial, and ultimately the intracellular space passes into the capillaries and compensates for the loss in circulating volume.

The inadequate perfusion of peripheral tissues has a number of effects:

1 *Lactic acidosis.* Because the supply of oxygen is inadequate for normal aerobic metabolism, a proportion of peripheral tissue metabolism becomes anaerobic, and in the absence of treatment of the shock state, a progressive metabolic (lactic) acidosis ensues.

2 *Myocardial depression.* For a number of reasons — hypoxia, acidosis and release of depressant substances from underperfused tissues — myocardial contractility is depressed and myocardial function and cardiac output deteriorate.

3 *Bacterial toxins.* It has been suggested that as a result of ischaemia the integrity of the intestinal mucosa is damaged, so that bacteria and bacterial toxins enter the blood stream and damage remote organs.

4 *The micro circulation.* Ultimately, as a result of persistent peripheral stagnation, alterations occur in blood flow characteristics and coagulation properties. Capillary stagnation leads to sludging of red cells and the capillary walls leak plasma into the interstitium. Blood clotting factors may be activated and intravascular coagulation occur.

Cardiogenic shock

Cardiogenic shock is a failure of peripheral perfusion but in this instance is due to failure of the central pump, i.e. the heart, to maintain an adequate output. The commonest cause is myocardial infarction but others include myocarditis, cardiac tamponade and the terminal stages of chronic heart failure.

Endotoxic shock

Endotoxic shock or septic shock is due to release of endotoxins most commonly from gram negative bacteria. These dilate the peripheral circulation producing hypotension, a decrease in venous return, a decrease in cardiac output and peripheral stagnation.

Other forms of shock

These include anaphylactic and vasovagal shock. In the former, arterial hypotension is due to histamine release following exposure to an antigen to which the patient is sensitized. It is often accompanied by bronchospasm and oedema, and is treated with adrenaline, steroids and intravenous fluids. Vasovagal shock is usually a temporary phenomenon due to an autonomic imbalance caused often by emotional upset. Profound peripheral vasodilatation is accompanied by bradycardia. Peripheral pooling of the circulating blood results in a drastic decrease in cardiac output, cerebral hypoperfusion results and the individual who is usually standing loses consciousness and falls to the floor. This is normally only momentary as cardiac output is restored by the supine position and normal autonomic control of the circulation is regained, cerebral perfusion returns to normal and the individual recovers.

TREATMENT OF SHOCK

Treatment is aimed at restoring the cardiac output and peripheral circulation to normal. The hypovolaemia is treated with intravenous fluids, the type of fluid depending on the nature of the deficit, the degree and timing of the deficit and what fluid is available. Blood loss should be replaced with whole blood, but most fit healthy individuals tolerate an acute loss of up to 10–15% of their circulating blood volume with little or no ill effect. With greater losses, balanced salt solutions (lactated Ringers, Hartmanns solution) or plasma expanders — dextran or starch gells — are satisfactory alternatives until compatible blood is available.

Vasopressors and vasodilators. The mainstay of shock treatment is the restoration of circulating blood volume and cardiac output by infusion of blood or fluids, but vasodilators may be necessary in some circumstances to open up the blood flow to those areas where it has been decreased by intense sympathetic vasoconstriction.

At one time it was considered that the objective of treating shock was to keep the blood pressure up, and to this end vasopressors such as metaraminol were administered. However, this results in a further decrease in blood supply to tissues which are already underperfused.

Steriods in pharmacological doses such as methylprednisolone 1–2 g have been associated with improvements in condition, probably because of improvement in myocardial contractility and a peripheral vasodilating effect. Steroids also prevent aggregation of blood elements and decrease the likelihood of embolus and thrombus formation in the stagnant peripheral vascular system.

Antibiotics are of obvious value in septic shock.

Bicarbonate is used to correct the metabolic acidosis.

Oxygen. In severe hypotension arterial oxygenation mechanisms within the lung — the relationships between ventilation and perfusion — are frequently disturbed resulting in hypoxaemia.

Cardiac inotropes. With a prolonged period of shock, myocardial function deteriorates and the heart may need a period of pharmacological support for which dopamine is probably the current drug of choice.

LATE COMPLICATIONS

Renal failure

After any period of hypotension the kidneys are at risk of ischaemic damage and failure. Measures should be taken to maintain urine output, such as ensuring adequate hydration, and possibly giving an osmotic or loop diuretic.

'Shock lung'

A further complication has come to light over the past 20 years with improvements in techniques of resuscitation and evacuation. Patients survive their initial injury, are successfully resuscitated and apparently on the way to recovery, but succumb later from 'shock lung'. This is seen when the victim has suffered from quite a severe shock episode. Some time — a few hours to a few days — after injury and resuscitation, his respiratory condition starts to deteriorate. He becomes tachypnoeic. His chest X-ray and his blood gases are initially relatively normal or he may be moderately hypoxaemic with a normal or low arterial carbon dioxide tension. Diffuse scattered infiltrates appear over both lung fields and these may then eventually coalesce to form a diffuse white infiltrate.

Measurements of pulmonary capillary wedge pressure — a measure of left ventricular filling pressure — have been normal, so the cause is something other than left-sided heart failure. The aetiology of this condition is still not entirely clear. Theories include damage to pulmonary capillaries from micro aggregate debris in stored blood, and for this reason all transfused blood should be passed through a fine pore filter before administration. The idea that clear fluid given during resuscitation and sequestered in the tissues may be remobilized into the circulation has been put forward, but in view of the normal left-sided filling pressures this is unlikely. However, if the pulmonary capillaries have been damaged, and therefore leak, it is possible that transfused fluid could finish up in the alveolar space and the pulmonary capillary wedge pressure still be normal. It is this latter factor — damage to pulmonary capillaries — that is considered to be the most likely cause of shock lung. Stasis and disintegration of blood elements, principally white cells, in the pulmonary circulation, with the resulting release of intracellular enzymes, are thought to damage the walls of the pulmonary capillaries and cause extravasation of fluid into the alveolar spaces. Treatment of shock lung consists of ventilatory support by means of intermittent positive pressure ventilation until the pathology resolves, taking prophylactic measures to prevent secondary pulmonary infection.

Chapter 15

Respiratory Support

DEFINITION OF RESPIRATORY FAILURE

Respiratory failure is defined in terms of the partial pressures of oxygen and carbon dioxide in arterial blood. The figures generally quoted are that respiratory failure is present when the oxygen tension is less than and/or the CO_2 tension is greater than 50–60 mmHg (6.5–8 kPa) with the patient breathing air. In terms of the blood gas results two sorts of respiratory failure are recognized:

1 hypoxaemic failure, when arterial oxygen desaturation is present but Pa_{CO_2} is normal or maybe slightly decreased;

2 ventilatory failure, when hypercarbia and hypoxaemia are present simultaneously.

Hypoxaemic respiratory failure

This is usually due to disturbances in ventilation/perfusion relationships in the lung, the most severe of which is shunting of blood through alveoli which are not ventilated due to collapse or consolidation. The lung is usually able to cope with this by an increase in ventilation to keep the Pa_{CO_2} normal. If the hypoxaemia is severe enough to stimulate respiration itself, Pa_{CO_2} may be lower than normal. If the lung pathology decreases compliance the work of breathing increases and the patient may eventually get exhausted. His respiratory muscles tire and ventilatory failure supervenes. Causes of the hypoxaemic type of respiratory failure include severe pulmonary infections and the adult respiratory distress syndrome.

Ventilatory failure

This occurs when alveolar ventilation is inadequate for gas exchange. Causes include central depression due to drug overdose, head injury or diseases of the nervous system (myasthenia gravis, Guillain – Barré syndrome), exhaustion from some acute conditions as described above or acute exacerbation of chronic chest disease.

MANAGEMENT OF RESPIRATORY FAILURE

Hypoxaemic respiratory failure may need only an increase in the inspired oxygen level to restore the Pao_2 to normal. This can be accomplished by a variety of methods — nasal prongs or a nasopharyngeal cannula will raise the inspired oxygen concentration (FIO_2) to 30%, or various types of oxygen mask are available whereby the FIO_2 can be elevated to 50–60% provided the patient will tolerate the mask. If this restores the blood gases to normal, and the patient is not getting exhausted, this, along with the definitive treatment of the cause of the respiratory failure — antibiotics, physiotherapy, humidification, etc. — may be all that is required. If, however, because of an increase in respiratory work the patient does get exhausted, $Paco_2$ starts to rise denoting the onset of ventilatory failure. The management of ventilatory failure consists essentially of supporting ventilation and maintaining gas exchange by means of intermittent positive pressure ventilation (IPPV) while the underlying condition is treated or resolves.

Respiratory support with intermittent positive pressure ventilation (IPPV)

Control of the patient's airway is gained using an endotracheal tube or by way of a tracheostomy and positive pressure applied intermittently to the airway inflating the lungs. Expiration occurs passively by virtue of the lungs' own elastic recoil. Instituting this procedure has the following implications.

Control of the airway

Control of the airway is initially with an endotracheal tube. If a patient is to be ventilated for longer than a few hours he is easier to nurse and, if ventilation is to continue while he is conscious, it is more comfortable for him if the tube is passed via the nose rather than the mouth, although this may cause necrosis of the alae nasae which is difficult to treat. Most people would perform a tracheostomy if IPPV has to be continued beyond 1–2 weeks. The argument against this is that a trachoestomy carries its own morbidity and mortality — displacement of the tube, erosion through the carotid artery, etc. — and has the later complication of tracheal stenosis which is serious.

Control of ventilation

Most patients initially tolerate IPPV very badly and have to be heavily sedated with narcotics — morphine, phenoperidine, etc — to allow it to be carried out effectively. There is a reluctance to fully paralyse a patient undergoing prolonged IPPV because in the event of a mishap, such as disconnection from the ventilator, the patient is left totally unable to breathe.

Control of secretions

A tube passed into the trachea makes the patient unable to cough and so unable to rid himself of respiratory secretions by the normal mechanisms. In respiratory failure these may be copious. The usual practice is to facilitate their aspiration with physiotherapy and intermittent hyperinflations of the lung, aspirating secretions from the trachea using a suitable catheter passed down the tracheostomy or endotracheal tube. Loss of the usual humidification mechanism of the nose and pharynx also means that tracheal and bronchial secretions dry out and are difficult or impossible to aspirate and may block the tracheostomy or endotracheal tube. All respiratory circuits connected to the trachea and bronchi for extended periods must contain some means of humidifying the inspired air.

Postural drainage and pressure areas

Heavily sedated or paralysed patients are unable to move and are in danger of developing hypostatic pneumonia and pressure sores. Patients on ventilators should preferably be nursed on their side and turned at regular intervals, i.e. about every 2 hours.

Effect of IPPV on the cardiovascular system

In normal circumstances, venous return to the heart is dependent on the muscle pump, negative intrathoracic pressure and the pressure in the venous side of the circulation — the resultant of blood volume and venous tone. During IPPV, the muscle pump is often abolished by heavy sedation or maybe even muscle relaxants, so that mean intrathoracic pressure is positive. Venous return is therefore dependent on compensatory venoconstrictor mechanisms. This does not normally cause problems, but in patients with some impairment of their sympathetic nervous system — such as the elderly, those on long term antihypertensive therapy, diabetics or patients who are hypovolaemic and already maximally compensated — it may do so. The problem is also exacerbated if the inspiratory phase in the ventilator cycle is unduly long, as this raises mean intrathoracic pressure even higher.

Carbon dioxide is a potent sympathetic stimulant. Patients who are retaining CO_2, either chronically or acutely, may be depending on this to maintain their blood pressure and cardiac output, and are in danger of dramatic falls in cardiac output and blood pressure if they are put onto IPPV and their Pa_{CO_2} is reduced to 'normal' levels immediately. In these circumstances Pa_{CO_2} should be reduced gradually.

Infection

Tracheostomies invariably become infected because of their position. As the normal protective mechanisms have been bypassed, the respiratory tract itself is also more liable to infection. Scrupulous attention should be paid to aseptic handling of suction catheters, etc.

Fluids and Feeding

Unconscious ventilated patients are unable to swallow and may have a paralytic ileus. Fluid requirements are given intravenously and, as the patient is heavily sedated, a urinary catheter is usually passed. If they are still unable to take anything by mouth after 2–3 days intravenous feeding is usually started. Very ill patients on IPPV do not tolerate enteral feeding well because of nausea, abdominal distention, vomiting, regurgitation and diarrhoea, but as their condition improves and they become conscious and co-operative, feeding via a nasogastric or nasoenteral tube may become feasible and is preferable to the intravenous route as it is more physiological, does not have the morbidity of intravenous feeding and is less expensive.

Monitoring

One of the aims of IPPV is to produce blood gas tensions within normal limits. With reliable and robust blood gas electrodes the effectiveness with which this aim is achieved is relatively easy to determine. In general the level of $Paco_2$ depends on ventilation and fresh gas flows into the ventilator circuitry. Arterial Pco_2 should be maintained at about 35 mmHg (6 kPa) and Pao_2 should be above 70 mmHg (9.3 kPa). Very low carbon dioxide tensions impair cardiac output and produce cerebral vasoconstriction, which in a head injury may to a certain degree be desirable, but in normal circumstances is not. Arterial Pco_2 levels much higher than this may stimulate the patients own respiratory drive and cause them to 'fight the ventilator'.

The maintenance of optimal blood gases for prolonged periods in a critically ill patient is easier if an indwelling intra arterial cannula is inserted to facilitate frequent arterial blood sampling.

Oxygenation

This depends on the appropriate matching of ventilation and perfusion. The most severe form of ventilation perfusion mismatch is the shunting of blood through collapsed or consolidated alveoli. Oxygenation of blood perfusing alveoli which are well perfused but badly ventilated can be imroved by increasing the oxygen concentration in the inspired air. Oxygen concentrations much above 50–60%, however, are toxic to lung tissue, so it is undesirable that FIO_2 should go above this level. Improvements in ventilation and oxygenation can be brought about by the application of positive pressure, usually of 5 or 10 cm of water, to the expiratory limb of the respiratory circuit to maintain these pressures in the patients respiratory tract at the end of expiration — positive end expiratory pressure (PEEP). This improves oxygenation by keeping open alveoli which are poorly ventilated and tending to collapse, and small airways which are tending to close in the latter half of expiration. This improvement in oxygenation allows Pao_2 levels to be maintained with a lower FIO_2. The disadvantage of the technique is that if the PEEP is transmitted to the pulmonary vascular bed (which with badly diseased lungs it very often is not), it effectively raises the mean intrathoracic pressure with its undesirable effect on venous return and cardiac output.

It is normal practice to monitor the ventilator settings — tidal volume, respiratory rate, inspired oxygen concentrations, inflation pressure and humidifier temperature.

Weaning from IPPV

Patients who have been ventilated for prolonged periods often experience difficulty in resuming independent spontaneous ventilation. This may be due to residual disease in the lung, decreased compliance and the increased work of breathing, but with prolonged periods of IPPV it is often due to a loss of muscular co-ordination and alterations in the pattern of respiratory drive. Spontaneous ventilation has to be re-learnt.

Common techniques are:

1   *Weaning*. IPPV is stopped for brief periods at regular intervals, e.g. 5 minutes in every hour, the length of time increasing as the patient gradually learns to cope.

2   *Triggering*. Many ventilators have a mechanism whereby the inspiratory phase of the respiratory cycle is 'triggered' by a minimal inspiratory effort on the part of the patient and reinforces this effort.

3   *Intermittent mandatory ventilation*. This is probably now the most popular method of getting a patient back to breathing on his own. The ventilator circuit is designed so that between 'mandatory ventilations' from the ventilator he is able to breath spontaneously through the circuitry. The frequency of mandatory ventilations is decreased gradually over a period as rapidly as the patient can tolerate, the limiting factors being the patient's comfort and the resulting change (or lack of change) in blood gases.

TRACHEOSTOMY

Tracheostomy carries its own morbidity and mortality and should not be undertaken lightly. It can be performed under local anaesthesia but is distressing for the patient, and is better done under a general anaesthetic with an anaesthetist in proper control of the airway.

Indications for tracheostomy are:

1 obstruction of the upper respiratory tract, e.g. neoplasm or glottic oedema;

2 to aid aspiration of respiratory secretions when coughing is ineffective, e.g. following a crush injury of the chest;

3 to separate the respiratory and digestive tracts and prevent pulmonary aspiration, e.g. with a bulbar palsy;

4 to make IPPV easier.

The complications of trachoesomy are:

1 *Infection.* This is almost inevitable in view of the site of the stoma.

2 *Obstruction* due to inspissated secretions and inadequate humidification or misplacement or dislodgement of the tracheostomy tube into the tissues of the neck.

3 *Haemorrhage.* The tube can ulcerate through the wall of the trachea into the innominate artery resulting in torrential haemorrhage.

4 *Surgical emphysema* due to air leaking into the tissues of the neck or a pneumothorax if the tracheostomy is performed too low.

5 *Tracheal stenosis* is a late complication and may require surgical repair.

Chapter 16

Cardiopulmonary Resuscitation

DEFINITION OF CARDIAC ARREST

The condition commonly called 'cardiac arrest' is defined as failure of the heart to provide an adequate cerebral circulation in the absence of irreversible disease. It should be noted that the definition is a mechanical one in that it relates to output and not to electrical activity, so on their own the ECG findings may be irrelevant. The other point to note is that resuscitative measures are appropriate in the 'absence of irreversible disease'. They are not appropriate when cardiac standstill is an inevitable outcome of the patient's illness such as disseminated malignant disease.

The signs of 'cardiac arrest' are:
1 loss of consciousness;
2 absent major pulses — carotid and femoral;
3 absent respiration;
4 fixed dilated pupils.

The diagnosis should be made on the first two of these criteria, as respiration may continue for up to a minute after the heart has stopped and likewise it may take up to a minute for the pupils to dilate. Consciousness is lost within 5–15 seconds of the cardiac output ceasing. Failure to institute effective cerebral oxygenation within 2–3 minutes results in irreversible brain damage and eventually 'brain death'.

IMMEDIATE ACTION

1 *Shout for help.* You will be unable to cope with this situation by yourself for very long.

2 *Thump the chest.* Occasionally, particularly in young fit people with a sound myocardium, the non specific stimulus of a sharp thump on the precordium may start the heart.
3 *Clear the airway* of vomit, false teeth or anything else that may be obstructing it.
4 *Institute artificial ventilation and external cardiac massage* It is not intended to discuss these procedures in detail but a few points should be made.

Intermittent Positive Pressure Ventilation (IPPV)

1 This will have to be mouth to mouth artificial ventilation in the first instance until an artificial aid such as a 'Brook Airway' or an 'Ambu Bag' and anaesthetic mask can be obtained.
2 The chest must be seen to move with each ventilation.
3 Do not attempt to intubate the patient unless you are absolutely certain of getting the endotracheal tube into the trachea. If the tube is inadvertently passed into the oesophagus and the stomach inflated, regurgitation will almost inevitably ensue with airway obstruction and the stomach contents will probably enter the trachea and lung.
4 If you are by yourself, then the ratio of one inflation of the lungs to four or five compressions of the heart is appropriate.

External Cardiac Massage (ECM)

The object of this procedure is to compress the heart between the sternum and the vertebral column thereby producing an artificial systole. The heel of one hand should be placed on the lower half of the sternum, the other hand over the dorsum of the first; keeping the elbows straight, and leaning over the patient so that the weight of the shoulders are directly above the hands, you should compress the sternum sharply through 3–5 cm 60–80 times/minute. A faster rate than this does not allow an adequate 'diastole' for the heart to fill. The older the patient is, the more rigid his thoracic cage, the harder it is to produce an adequate cardiac output, the more likely you are to fracture ribs or sternum and to damage other organs such as liver, kidney, spleen or lungs. Avoid spreading your hands and fingers over the rib cage as this will also increase the chance of breaking ribs. If the cardiac compression is adequate, a pressure wave should be palpable in the femoral artery. When help arrives, get them to continue the cardiac massage, at least initially as this is the most tiring, while you continue with the ventilation.

It has been the practice in the past to stop the ECM momentarily every four or five compressions while the lungs are ventilated. However, recent work has suggested that external cardiac massage may work, not by compressing the heart between the sternum and the vertebral bodies, but merely by raising the intrathoracic pressure and so compresing the heart from all round. In view of this it is now also accepted practice to continue ECM throughout ventilation. Precisely what the best technique is has not yet been entirely settled. Done efficiently artificial ventilation and external cardiac massage should provide oxygenation and a cardiac output sufficient to keep the brain alive until definitive treatment for the arrest can be instituted and spontaneous heart action restored.

Signs that circulation and ventilation are adequate are:
1   improvement in colour;
2   pupils constrict;
3   spontaneous ventilation may return;
4   level of consciousness may improve.

USE OF EQUIPMENT

If the arrest has occurred outside hospital the patient should be transferred to hospital and external cardiac massage and intermittent positive pressure ventilation continued during the journey. If the arrest has occurred in hospital all the equipment required for definitive treatment can be brought to the patient.

With the arrival of experienced help and the appropriate equipment the priorities are as follows.

Secure the airway

This essentially means passing a cuffed endotracheal tube by an individual skilled in that procedure and instituting positive pressure ventilation with pure oxygen and an appropriate means of delivering it such an anaesthetic reservoir bag or an 'Ambu Bag'.

Establish an intravenous line

This is for drug administration. This can be difficult in a cold collapsed pulseless patient but if there are no accessible peripheral veins the external jugular usually provides a suitable site and in these circumstances is not difficult to get into even for the relatively inexperienced.

Establish an electrocardiograph

This is to determine the state of the myocardium. The ECG will show one of two basic pictures:
1   asystole;
2   ventricular fibrillation.

Asystole

The ECG picture of this condition is a flat tracing. Infrequent wide bizarre QRS complexes should be interpreted as asystole and treated as such.

Ventricular fibrillation

This may be 'coarse' or 'fine'. Fine fibrillation is when the myofibrils of the cardiac muscle are contracting separately and asychronously. Its ECG characteristics are low voltage high frequency changes. This is a difficult form of fibrillation to convert to sinus rhythm. Coarse fibrillation occurs when muscle fibres are contracting in groups so there is some semblance of synchronous action. Its characteristics are low frequency high voltage variations in the ECG tracing. With many fibres contracting together it is an easier form of fibrillation to convert to sinus rhythm than fine fibrillation.

DEFINITIVE TREATMENT OF A CARDIAC ARREST

Treatment of the metabolic acidosis

Any patient in a state of circulatory arrest will develop a metabolic acidosis due to anaerobic metabolism continuing in the peripheral tissues. Ideally arterial blood should be taken, acid base status determined immediately and the appropriate amount of sodium bicarbonate administered, usually as an 8.4% solution which contains 1 mmol/ml. In practice this is rarely possible. If 100–200 mmol of NaHCO$_3$ is given empirically and a further 50 mmol every 15 minutes for the duration of the arrest, this should effectively treat the major part of the acidosis and in itself is unlikely to produce any abnormality.

The dangers of giving excessive quantities of bicarbonate are the large sodium load (1 mmol/ml) in the presence of an already compromised circulation, and the danger of inducing a metabolic alkalosis which may have an adverse effect on cardiac output should the circulation be restored.

Treatment of asystole

This has traditionally been with drugs which stimulate the myocardium — adrenaline 10 ml of 1 in 10,000 calcium salts (chloride or gluconate) 1 g (10 ml of a 10% solution) or isoprenaline 0.2 mg in 10 ml saline. However, recent work has shown that these patients already have very high levels of blood catecholamines, and to give additional myocardial stimulants may be pointless. Broadly two sorts of asystole are recognized: in one the myocardium is dead and no amount of stimulant drugs will cure that, and in the other asystole is present because of very high levels of cholinergic (vagal) activity. It has been suggested that in asystole atropine should be the first drug of choice given in doses of 1.2 mg and repeated as often as necessary.

It should also be remembered that calcium salts given into an infusion containing sodium bicarbonate will cause a precipitation of calcium carbonate.

Treatment of ventricular fibrillation

Treatment of ventricular fibrillation (VF) is with DC countershock using an external defibrillator. The paddles of the instrument are placed along the electrical axis of the heart one at the base and one at the apex. A DC shock of 200 joules is tried first and if ineffective is repeated with 50 joule increments until shocks of 400 joules are administered. The paddle should be spread liberally with conduction electrode jelly to ensure that

1   the shock is transmitted to the patient's heart, and that

2 the patient is not burnt. Fine VF is hard to convert to sinus rhythm but if treated with cardiac stimulants (calcium salts, isoprenaline, adrenaline) may convert to coarse fibrillation.

If it proves impossible to convert coarse fibrillation to sinus rhythm, or if as soon as sinus rhythm is restored it reverts to VF, it may be necessary to administer drugs to decrease myocardial irritability such as lignocaine, a beta-blocker or one of the calcium antagonists. The problem with administering these agents is that they are myocardial depressants and can cause asystole or depress cardiac output if spontaneous cardiac action is restored.

ON RESTORATION OF SINUS RHYTHM AND A SPONTANEOUS CARDIAC OUTPUT

Cardiac excitability

The heart may still be in an irritable excitable state. Ventricular ectopic beats may be seen: these may be multifocal and the heart's action may revert back to ventricular fibrillation after sinus rhythm has been restored. The excitability again may be treated with drugs that depress myocardial excitability — such as lignocaine, beta-blockers, etc.

Support of tissues sensitive to hypoxia

Because of the hypoxic insult and possibly also as a result of the initial insult (e.g. myocardial infarction) myocardial function on restoration of sinus rhythm may be deficient and some temporary form of myocardial support may be necessary, either pharmacological (dopamine, isoprenaline or adrenaline) or mechanical (e.g. intra-aortic balloon pump). The hypoxia caused by the arrest may cause renal and cerebral damage. Vigorous efforts should be made to restore renal function as quickly as possible by restoring blood pressure and by the use of osmotic diuretics such as mannitol. Steps can be taken to prevent cerebral oedema by the use of IPPV, steroids and osmotic diuretics.

WHEN TO ABANDON RESUSCITATION

The question does arise as to when resuscitation attempts should be abandoned as futile. In a patient with fixed dilated pupils who has been in asystole for half an hour there is little point in continuing. The problems arise in patients who are in ventricular fibrillation (which implies their heart is salvageable) but with fixed dilated pupils (which implies their brain probably is not), or in asystole with normal pupils possibly even reacting to light, the implication being that the brain is functioning but the heart is unlikely to function again.

Chapter 17

Head Injury

Head injury is a major problem which has enormous social consequences. One per cent of all deaths in Britain are due to head injury and this represents 25% of all deaths from trauma. The largest single group is due to road traffic accidents which account for 6000 deaths a year in the UK — half of these are associated with head injury. The acute management of head injury is critical and may well determine the eventual outcome — from death, through varying grades of central nervous malfunction with epilepsy, to apparent normality.

PATHOLOGY

The brain can be damaged in many ways. The initial trauma can damage the brain underlying the area of impact, by 'contracoup', by displacement of a skull fracture, by causing major intracranial haemorrhage and by inducing diffuse petechial haemorrhages. Secondary brain damage can occur with a rise in intracranial pressure due either to intracranial bleeding, or oedema, or to the effects of hypotension or cardiorespiratory arrest. This secondary brain damage is due to ischaemia or hypoxia.

PRINCIPLES OF MANAGEMENT

The acute management of the patient with a head injury is designed to avoid brain damage by maintaining optimal oxygenation of brain by adequate perfusion with oxygenated blood.

The airway

All unconscious or semiconscious patients are liable to develop systemic hypoxia due to airway obstruction. Airway obstruction, together with coughing and straining, causes a potentially dangerous rise in intracranial pressure (ICP). The commonest obstruction is the tongue, but aspiration of gastric contents or other foreign material including blood and teeth is also common, especially if the fracture involves the base of the skull. Although protection of the airway is the first priority, difficulties may arise because of suspected spinal injuries. It could be hazardous to move the patient into a lateral position to protect against aspiration, as this could result in spinal cord compression. Careful endotracheal intubation with a cuffed tube should be performed as soon as possible by someone skilled in this manoeuvre.

Ventilation

In a severe head injury, ventilation is usually inadequate or absent and must be provided initially with a mask and bag until endotracheal intubation allows the use of a mechanical ventilator.

Cardiovascular collapse

Cerebral perfusion depends on blood pressure. Cardiovascular collapse can be secondary to hypovolaemia and multiple injuries as well as brain stem trauma; one third of severe head injuries have other associated injuries. Both tachycardia and bradycardia can occur and require corrective treatment.

Assessment of head injury

The following physical signs should be used to assess the severity of brain damage:
1 *Level of consciousness*: response to verbal commands or response to painful stimuli including vocalization, eye opening or eye movements.
2 *Pupillary signs*: size and reaction to light.
3 *Brain stem activity*: respiratory pattern, heart rate, blood pressure, core temperature.
4 *Peripheral neurological examination*: muscle tone, spontaneous activity, convulsions.

Further information will be obtained from X-ray examinations of the skull, chest and cervical spine. Ultrasonic techniques are used to detect midline shift, although much more information is provided by computerized tomography (CT scan).

Monitoring progress

Though an initial assessment is important, of greater prognostic value is a record of change. Many centres use a 'coma scale' which is a numerical expression of the neurological state, and includes verbal and motor response, eye signs, etc. In a severe head injury, the coma scale variables may be difficult to interpret as the patient will usually be ventilated and may be receiving muscle relaxants and analgesics.

During the early post-traumatic period, one of the major problems is the development of cerebral oedema which causes a rise in ICP, thereby reducing the cerebral perfusion pressure and cerebral perfusion. ICP monitoring is used in many centres especially in the first 3 days after injury, to detect the early rise in pressure indicating the development of oedema. ICP monitoring requires a burr hole and placement of a catheter or equivalent fluid-filled system connected to a transducer. Control of ICP associated with oedema is achieved by hyperventilation (hypocapnia causes cerebral vasoconstriction and a reduction of the CSF volume). Other methods include avoidance of hypotension, osmotic diuresis with mannitol (0.3 g/kg initially) and hypnotic infusion using a barbiturate or one of the newer induction agents.

Brain death

One of the dilemmas of the modern treatment of head injury using ventilation of the lungs is the brain death of a victim with a viable and even healthy body. The diagnosis of brain death can only be made after the event, and with it comes the implied need to discontinue treatment by turning off the ventilator and allowing the victim's body to die. This is now further complicated by renal transplantation which requires the kidneys to be removed from a 'living' body while they are still fully oxygenated, and before the ventilation is discontinued. Brain death can never be completely proved but only inferred from the results of brain function tests which include:

1   absence of ventilation (with a Pco_2 greater than 7.5 kPa),
2   absence of gag and tracheal reflexes;
3   absence of motor response to painful stimuli;
4   absence of eye reflex response to ice-cold water in the external auditory canal.

Other tests, such as a flat electroencephalogram (EEG) and absence of cerebral perfusion with carotid angiography, are not universally accepted to be necessary. More important than these extra tests are the prerequisites before brain tests are performed. It is essential that the patient is not receiving CNS depressant drugs or muscle relaxants and has a body temperature greater than 35°C. The most critical prerequisite, however, is a knowledge of the likely severity and type of brain damage which has occurred.

Chapter 18

Management of Acute Poisoning

The majority of severely poisoned patients are admitted through the casualty department. The diagnosis is often in doubt as it is particularly difficult to differentiate the many causes of coma, and even before coma occurs there are often major behavioural changes which hinder history taking. Help from relatives will often assist in establishing a working diagnosis which gives the chemical pathologist and toxicologist a better chance of identifying the cause.

EMERGENCY MANAGEMENT

Three-quarters of poisoned patients are in little danger and treatment need only be symptomatic; the rest, however, may be in a life-threatening situation.

Emergency management includes:
1 removal from contact with poison;
2 assessment of vital signs especially respiration and heart beat;
3 clearing and protecting the airway by positioning or intubating the trachea to avoid aspiration of gastric contents;
4 providing artificial respiration when necessary;
5 moving to hospital.

Emergency drug treatment can include nalaxone for suspected opioid poisoning (small pupils, slow deep respiration), atropine for organophosphorous poisoning, and dicobalt edetate for cyanide. Oxygen should always be administered to unconscious and respiratorily embarrassed patients when available.

Not only is the identity of the chemical poison and the quantity of ingestion of importance, but also the time interval.

Poisons having a delayed action include the amanita fungi, paracetamol and paraquat — the tragedy with some of these late onset poisons is the comparative impotence of medical treatment even when it is administered to an initially conscious patient.

CLINICAL SIGNS

Cardiovascular changes

The most important cardiovascular signs include arrhythmias and hypotension, and either or both may proceed to cardiac arrest. Hypotension is particularly common and is due both to inappropriate peripheral vasodilatation and direct myocardial depression. Peripheral vascular changes may be due to direct action of drugs or autonomic failure as with beta-adrenergic antagonists. Persistent hypotension results in hypoxic damage to the brain, liver and kidneys, and will compound with the deleterious effects of the chemical poison.

The treatment of hypotension includes the administration of i.v. fluids via an adequate catheter whilst monitoring the urine output and central venous pressure. Oxygen therapy will help in the short term and inotropes will usually improve both the cardiac and renal outputs.

Neurological signs

Central nervous depression may occur as a direct effect of a drug overdose such as one of the benzodiazepines, or secondarily due to hypoxia, hypoglycaemia, hypocalcaemia or other metabolic disturbance. An important difference is the susceptibility of the hypoxic brain to develop increased and abnormal activity followed by convulsions. Some drugs including the tricyclic antidepressants induce convulsions directly.

The important neurological signs to elicit and record include level of consciousness, extrapyramidal movements, spontaneous activity, size of pupils, pupillary reflexes, tendon jerks and plantar responses. Respiratory distress and hypotension may indirectly reflect central nervous depression. A fall in body core temperature may be due to direct hypothalamic depression, or to the action of the drug on the skin blood vessels or on the peripheral autonomic nervous system influencing the sweating reflex activity.

Respiration

Respiratory complications are responsible for most deaths from poisoning. Aspiration of gastric contents frequently leads to either Mendelson's syndrome or adult respiratory distress syndrome (ARDS). Aspiration is always likely when respiratory reflexes are depressed and the patient is not in a semiprone (coma) position.

Coma itself predispses to airway obstruction due to tongue impaction in the oropharynx.

Central depression results in failure of respiratory drive and absence of hypercarbic stimulation of the respiratory centre. Peripheral muscle and nerve toxins can cause a curare-like muscle paralysis with a restrictive type of respiratory failure. The treatment of all these complications is logical, namely, to establish a clear airway using an endotracheal tube and to ventilate the lungs with an enriched oxygen gas mixture. Bronchoscopy and lavage of the bronchial tree with normal saline often lessens the lung damage following aspiration.

Kidney

Pre-renal failure may result from hypotension.

Renal parenchymal failure, however, can occur as a direct result of poisons on glomerular and tubular cells, for example paracetamol.

Post-renal failure may be due to obstruction of tubules with myoglobin, following rhabdomyolysis, or oxalate, after ethylene glycol ingestion.

Liver failure

This often occurs in conjunction with renal failure as in paracetamol poisoning or with amanita phalloides. Certain anaesthetics, or related compounds, such as carbon tetrachloride are well known hepatotoxins.

DIAGNOSIS OF THE CAUSE

The initial assessment must include smelling the breath, saving urine, vomitus or gastric aspirates, and faeces for chemical analysis, and recording carefully the state of consciousness, respiration, cardiovascular and renal function. These 'base line' observations prove to be invaluable in detecting trends as physical status deteriorates.

TREATMENT

The reader is referred to an excellent series of articles by various authors in the *British Medical Journal* in the summer of 1984 for details of specific agents. Local drug information units are often very helpful together with a local or a national Poison's Bureau.

The types of treatment employed are designed:

1   to delay or arrest absorption from the gut (such as gastric lavage);

2   to increase the rate of removal from the body (such as haemodialysis and diuresis);

3   to attempt to nullify the effect of the poison in the body (such as chelating agents).

Chapter 19

Intensive Care

The modern concept of intensive care originated in specialist high-dependency areas created to care for seriously ill patients, such as those recovering from cardiac surgery, those undergoing haemodialysis, or patients suffering from respiratory failure or from severe neurological disease affecting their level of consciousness or their ability to breath. Separate coronary, renal and neurological units have persisted in larger institutions but most district general hospitals provide a general intensive care service based on a purpose built unit.

The more common categories of patients admitted to intensive care are those who require artificial ventilation of the lungs, those needing a level of monitoring, particularly invasive monitoring, which would be unrealistic or dangerous on a general ward, those who need intensive nursing, such as the deeply unconscious and patients with multiple trauma and multiple organ failure.

ORGANIZATION

The need for intensive care in a typical district general hospital is estimated to be around 1–2% of all acute beds, as a higher figure results in an unacceptably low bed occupancy. It is also considered uneconomic to have an intensive care unit (ICU) smaller than six beds. The smallest hospital which would justify an ICU would therefore have a bed complement in the region of 300–400.

BEDSPACE

Each bed requires sufficient floor space, usually twice as much as on an ordinary ward, to accommodate bulky machinery —

ventilators, infusion pumps, etc. Each bedspace is supplied with multiple electrical outlets, piped gases (oxygen, nitrous oxide and air) and suction.

MONITORING EQUIPMENT

The degree of monitoring required for any patient obviously depends upon the severity of his illness, but basic monitoring facilities would include ECG with electronically derived heart rate, two pressure channels and two temperature channels.

STORAGE SPACE

Because of the large amount of bulky equipment, such as ventilators and haemodialysis machines, a large storage area is required and the conventional view is that storage space should be the same size as the total bed area.

ADDITIONAL FACILITIES

In addition there should be a sitting/tea room for medical and nursing staff and ideally a bedroom for a resident member of the medical staff. There should also be rooms for patients' visitors to wait in and to be interviewed in, and ideally accommodation within the hospital for them to stay overnight if necessary. There are of course the usual needs for sluice, kitchen, office, linen cupboards, etc.

MEDICAL STAFF

Most intensive care units are run by consultants who have trained primarily in one of the medical or surgical specialties and have a special interest in ICU. They have usually devoted only a part of their training period to intensive care. At the moment there are few specialist intensivists in the UK, but in the USA, Europe and Australia, where there are specialist training programmes in ICU, many individuals devote all their time to ICU work. In the UK a preponderance of the consultants running intensive care units are anaesthetists. This is an historical association because of the importance of ventilatory support in the treatment of many of the patients, but the care of the critically ill also demands a familiarity with medicine, surgery and resuscitation as well as physiology and pharmacology. No one doctor can be expected to be an expert in all these fields and it is normal practice to consult appropriate specialists when necessary. Many intensive care units have routine visits from, for example, bacteriologists, chemical pathologists and radiologists.

Policies about who manages the patient vary. In some units the consultant in charge has responsibility for all aspects of management, in others the admitting firm maintains responsibility, the consultant in charge of ICU having principally an administrative role. Junior members of the medical staff deal with the minute to minute problems and ideally should be present on the ward at all times and that includes sleeping there.

NURSING STAFF

High staffing levels of specially trained nurses are probably the most important part of intensive care and there should be at least one nurse by each bedside at all times. This means three nurses per patient for a 24 hour cover. When holidays and time off are considered, the ratio of total nurses per bed comes to about five or six.

PATIENT MANAGEMENT

Details of the various therapeutic and supportive techniques in common use on intensive care — respiratory support, cardiovascular monitoring, resuscitation, treatment of 'shock', management of head injuries, etc. — are dealt with elsewhere in this volume. Patients who are critically ill for prolonged periods and unable to take anything by mouth have to be fed either intravenously or fed enterally by means of a tube passed into the stomach or small bowel. Intravenous feeding is usually with solutions of glucose, fat and amino acids, and enteral feeding is now commonly undertaken using commercially available preparations either dripped into the stomach or small bowel by gravity or infused using a special pump. Patients on intensive care for longer than a couple of days usually have to be fed artificially, but a detailed discussion of artificial feeding techniques is beyond the scope of this book.

PSYCHOLOGICAL ASPECTS

Patients are on intensive care for varying periods of time. Many will spend only one night there following a major operation, others may be ventilated artificially for days or weeks or even months. Some may be fully conscious and aware of their surroundings, others heavily sedated and apparently oblivious to what is going on. It is important for all concerned with the provision of intensive care to appreciate that many apparently unconscious patients are actually aware of their surroundings. All patients, including the unconscious, should be kept informed verbally of what is happening to them, even if they are apparently unresponsive, and warned before procedures such as endotracheal suction are performed. Likewise relatives must be dealt with sympathetically and kept informed of developments.

Many patients recovering from a period on intensive care are unable to remember anything of the experience. Others remember hallucinatory phenomena, sensations of depersonalization, etc. There is reason to believe that these psychological disturbances may be related to disorientation in time and space resulting from the monotony of the environment and of the treatment. This particularly applies to patients undergoing long periods of heavy sedation used to facilitate intermittent positive pressure ventilation.

Chapter 20

Paediatric Anaesthesia

For the purpose of anaesthesia and surgery the paediatric population must not be regarded as small adults although they obviously do come to resemble adults as they get older. The problems of paediatric anaesthesia are exemplified by the problems of anaesthesia in the neonate.

PROBLEMS IN NEONATAL ANAESTHESIA

Factors that give rise to problems in neonatal anaesthesia are:
1 *Large surface area/volume ratio* with consequent increased heat and fluid loss. There is a danger of hypothermia due to the limited capacity of the thermoregulatory mechanisms in relation to the large surface area.
2 *Large tongue* in relation to the size of the mouth, but as babies are obligatory nose breathers this normally has little relevance unless there is choanal atresia.
3 *Poor respiratory reserve.* Resistance to laminar flow through parallel sided tubes such as the trachea and bronchi are a function of the fourth power of the radius (r^4), so the narrow air passages in the child have a disproportionately large effect on the work of breathing and the presence of even small amounts of secretions may induce turbulent flow and increase resistance to airflow. The ribs of the newborn are more horizontal than those of the adult or older child. The 'bucket handle' movement of ventilation is therefore virtually absent, so there is reduced inspiratory reserve capacity. In addition there is evidence that airways in the base of the lung close during quiet respiration, so there is a tendency to hypoxaemia.

4 *The liver.* The liver's enzyme systems are immature and unable to metabolize drugs as efficiently as the adult or older child.

5 *Neuromuscular transmission* in the newborn is also immature and the neonate is abnormally sensitive to non-depolarizing muscle relaxants.

The factors outlined above have a direct bearing on anaesthesia for the newborn:

Because of the dangers of hypothermia neonates should be transferred to the operating theatre in an incubator and active steps taken to prevent heat loss during induction of anaesthesia and during the operation, i.e. a warming blanket should be used and limbs and non-operated parts kept well insulated and the theatre temperature raised as high as is compatible with the comfort of the staff.

Because of the reduced respiratory reserve neonates should be ventilated and not allowed to breathe spontaneously. Uncuffed parallel sided endotracheal tubes only are used. The cricoid ring has the smallest diameter of any part of the upper respiratory tract so there is no need to use a cuffed endotracheal tube.

With the large tongue and edentulous mouth it is generally easier to use a straight bladed laryngoscope for intubation than a curved one. This is placed into the oesophagus and withdrawn slowly until the larynx comes into view, the blade therefore lying posterior to the epiglottis and actively lifting it up rather than pulling it forward as is done with the curved bladed instrument.

The endotracheal tube that is passed should fit loosely enough into the trachea to allow a small leak around the side to avoid the dangers of damaging the tracheal mucosa. Some paediatric anaesthetists pack the mouth lightly with lubricated gauze to help steady the tube in place.

PAEDIATRIC ANAESTHETIC APPARATUS

There are a number of different types of paediatric anaesthetic apparatus available. It is your responsibility to acquaint yourself with the type in common use in your own hospital. They are, however, all designed with the following principles in mind:

1 minimizing dead space, and
2 minimizing expiratory resistance and the work of breathing.

The use of adult sized apparatus in neonates and young children, with its large dead space in relation to a normal neonatal or infant tidal volume, would involve a significant amount of rebreathing, resulting in carbon dioxide retention and possibly even hypoxia. For this reason face masks are specially designed to fit flush on the face. Because of the diminished respiratory reserve and the already increased work of breathing, there are usually no expiratory valves on paediatric anaesthetic apparatus so that the work of breathing is minimized. Rebreathing is avoided by the design of the apparatus and the choice of appropriate gas flows.

PREMEDICATION

For children up to the age of 6–12 months it is common practice to give no premedication or maybe only intramuscular atropine to dry up secretions. This is particularly relevant in a group with narrow air passages as discussed earlier. Atropine should not be given to a child with a fever because of the dangers of inhibiting sweating and producing hyperpyrexia. In the older child views on premedication differ. Some would argue that if a child is dealt with sympathetically and his confidence is gained by the nursing and medical staff there should be no need for heavy opiate sedation, particularly if it involves a painful intramuscular injection. Others would argue that the benefits of having a quiet sedated child outweigh the pain and tribulations of administering the injection. Many anaesthetists use a non-opiate sedative such as trimeprazine or promethazine given orally 1–2 hours pre-operatively.

INDUCTION OF ANAESTHESIA

Views also differ over the desirability of intravenous induction as against inhalational. The occasional paediatric anaesthetist often feels safer administering a rapidly acting inhalational agent such as cyclopropane or halothane than trying to find a tiny vein in a struggling child. The skilled practitioner may prefer intravenous induction with a predetermined dose calculated from the patient's weight.

MAINTENANCE OF ANAESTHESIA

Certainly in the neonate and younger child, because of the relatively poor respiratory function most paediatric anaesthetists would choose to ventilate, usually by hand, rather than allow the child to breath spontaneously. Techniques of maintaining anaesthesia are much the same as in the adult — muscle relaxants, inhalational agent, intravenous opiates, doses being adjusted to body size. However, as neuromuscular transmission mechanisms in the neonate are immature, they are particularly sensitive to non-depolarizing muscle relaxants. Their immature liver enzymes also degrade narcotics poorly. Care has to be taken in the neonate in administering both these types of drug.

COMMON OPERATIONS

Many paediatric operations, such as insertion of ventricular shunts, repair of hare lip, etc., are highly specialized and carried out mostly in specialized referral units. There are two operations, though, which are done routinely and very frequently in most district general hospitals. Both have their problems.

Tonsillectomy and adenoidectomy

This is a relatively short routine procedure. The problems occur if the tonsillar bed bleeds post-operatively, when the consequences are potentially disastrous. The child that then has to be anaesthetized to stop this haemorrhage
1   is hypovolaemic,
2   has a stomach full of blood, so is in danger of vomiting and regurgitation, and
3   will have blood clots in the mouth and pharynx, which may obstruct respiration and make the passage of an endotracheal tube difficult after induction of anaesthesia.

Circumcision

Circumcision and a number of other operations around the groin such as hernia and orchidopexy are carried out frequently. The surgery is distressing and painful. Effective postoperative analgesia can be obtained quite easily in children using local anaesthetic techniques — injection of local anaesthetic through the caudal hiatus of the sacrum for any operation in the groin, or blockade of the dorsal nerves of the penis by injection of a small quantity of local anaesthetic at the base of the organ before circumcision provides very satisfactory analgesia for several hours particularly if bupivacaine is used.

Chapter 21

Obstetric Anaesthesia and Analgesia

ANATOMY AND PHYSIOLOGY

The sensory inervation of the body of the uterus comes from the spinal cord at the level of T11–12 but may involve T10 or L1. Innervation of the cervix, the lower segment of the uterus and the birth canal is from S2, 3 and 4. Special features of maternal physiology which affect anaesthetic management are largely those due to the presence of a large mass occupying most of the abdominal cavity. Lung volumes decrease; the diaphragm is elevated and splinted and respiratory efficiency impaired and there may be some difficulty in breathing particularly when lying flat. High progesterone levels during pregnancy stimulate respiration so the pregnant woman normally has a $Paco_2$ of about 32 mmHg.

When supine the uterus tends to obstruct the inferior vena cava and impedes the return of blood to the heart. In most people there are adequate collateral channels for blood to return to the heart via the system of veins around the vertebral column. In some individuals these collateral channels are absent or inadequate, and assumption of the supine position results in a precipitous drop in cardiac output and blood pressure and a sensation of 'feeling faint' — the so-called supine hypotensive syndrome. This is avoided if the patient lies on her side and caval compression is relieved.

The junction of the uterine and placental circulations represents a barrier which partially obstructs the passage of drugs and metabolites into the foetal circulation. The placental circulation is also affected by drugs administered to the mother such as vasoconstrictors and is sensitive to maternal blood gas/ acid base status.

OBSTETRIC ANALGESIA

Systemic analgesics

Early labour presents more as mild discomfort than severe pain, but when labour becomes established and the pain severe, powerful analgesia is required and the traditional narcotic analgesic is usually pethidine. The disadvantage is the respiratory depression it can produce in the newborn child. A narcotic analgesic should not be administered within 4–6 hours of the birth — a prerequisite which unfortunately it is not always possible to guarantee.

Inhalational analgesia

In the latter part of the first stage of labour and throughout the second stage the traditional method of analgesia has been the use of inhalational anaesthetic agents in subanaesthetic doses.

Entonox, probably the commest inhalational analgesic in use today, is a mixture of 50% oxygen and 50% nitrous oxide. Its advantages are that being relatively insoluble it acts quickly, is not cumulative and the 50% oxygen ensures the foetus is well oxygenated.

Trichlorethylene used with air in concentrations of 0.35 or 0.5% was a popular inhalational analgesic agent before Entonox. Being a very soluble vapour its onset of action is slower than Entonox, and it is cumulative in the tissues so can cause drowsiness. It still has a place in circumstances where there are problems with the supply of Entonox cylinders, such as in isolated communities.

Methoxyflurane, like trichlorethylene is a very soluble agent. It is delivered in concentrations of 0.35% in air. Its popularity has declined because of the renal problems associated with its use.

Uterine contractions and labour pains

Because of their cumulative characteristics the analgesic effects of trichlorethylene and methoxyflurane persist between labour pains. The same is not true for Entonox because of its relative insolubility, so for effective analgesia inhalation has to start before the pain becomes appreciable in order to give the agent time to work. The early part of a uterine contraction is usually painless so it is common practice to start inhaling the Entonox at the start of the contraction prior to the onset of the pain.

Epidural local analgesia

Since the development of the long acting amide anaesthetic bupivacaine, and since in the UK the English National Board gave permission for 'top ups' of epidural local anaesthesia to be given by midwives, this form of analgesia using an epidural cannula has become fairly common practice. Its main advantage is that the mother requires no narcotic analgesic, so the foetus is free of the depressant effects that narcotics cause. If an epidural works satisfactorily, the mother is completely free of pain.

The disadvantages of epidural analgesia are that it requires some degree of training and skill to insert an epidural cannula and to be able to maintain satisfactory analgesia. It also impairs the activity of the sympathetic nervous system, so hypotension, particularly in patients prone to the supine hypotensive syndrome, can be a serious problem. Hypotension is usually offset by the administration of intravenous fluids in the form of a balanced salt solution (0.5–1 litre) or a plasma expander. If vasopressors have to be used they should be of a type that do not cause constriction of the placental circulation. Ephedrine is the customary drug of choice.

The strength of local anaesthetic solution is chosen to produce sensory blockade with minimal motor block. If perineal sensation (S2, 3 and 4) is abolished completely and particularly if motor block occurs, the mother loses the desire (and the ability) to push. In the second stage she may then fail to expel the foetus by her own efforts making a forceps delivery necessary. Epidural analgesia carries its own morbidity and mortality.

ANAESTHESIA FOR OPERATIVE OBSTETRICS

Anaesthesia may be required for caesarian section or for any invasive procedure such as a high forceps delivery or removal of a retained placenta. These procedures can be carried out under epidural (or spinal) anaesthesia, and because of the dangers of anaesthesia in the obstetric patient this is preferable. If the mother already has an epidural cannula in place for labour, all that is required is to ensure that the epidural blockade is of adequate extent and intensity for the procedure to be carried out.

General anaesthesia

The problems associated with general anaesthesia in the parturient woman are as outlined in the introduction to this chapter, i.e. the supine hypotensive syndrome, the impairment of ventilation and the ability of depressant drugs to cross the placenta. In addition the woman in labour frequently has, for a variety of reasons — hormonal, mechanical and pharmacological — a delayed gastric emptying time. She must be assumed to have a full stomach and be in danger of vomiting, regurgitation and inhalation of stomach contents. All precautions must be taken against this happening, the most dangerous periods being on induction and recovery from anaesthesia.

Mendelson's syndrome

Mendelson's syndrome or aspiration pneumonia is caused by aspiration of gastric contents into the respiratory tree, and is characterized by severe bronchospasm, and diffuse pulmonary consolidation, resulting in pulmonary shunt and cyanosis. This is worse if the stomach contents have a low pH, and it is now routine practice on most obstetric units to administer regular prophylactic doses of antacids (such as magnesium trisilicate) to raise the gastric pH so that if the patient does have a general anaesthetic, regurgitates and aspirates, the effects of the stomach contents on the lung tissue is lessened.

Premedication

Premedication is usually with atropine alone and frequently given on induction. Any sedative or narcotic drug may cross the placenta and depress the foetus.

When supine the mother should lie on a wedge which tilts her pelvis to the left. This minimizes the effect of the uterus compressing the inferior vena cava and can be removed after the baby has been delivered. Haemorrhage is an ever present danger with caesarian section, so a secure intravenous line with a large cannula must be set up before induction and blood must be cross-matched and immediately available, although in an emergency this may not always be possible.

Induction

The patient is pre-oxygenated and suction is immediately to hand. Depending on the anaesthetist's preference, cricoid pressure may be applied or the patient may be intubated on her side as a precaution against regurgitation and vomiting. Induction is usually with a minimal dose of induction agent given as a bolus, followed by a muscle relaxant to allow intubation. This is usually suxamethonium because of its rapid action. A longer acting non-depolarizing agent is given when the effect of suxamethonium has worn off. Between induction and delivery the priorities are to maintain muscle relaxation and analgesia in the mother but cause as little disturbance to the foetus as possible. The mother must be kept well oxygenated with a high inspired oxygen and ventilated to maintain arterial P_{CO_2} at normal levels and avoid placental vasoconstriction. Because the general anaesthetic is very light, it is common practice to supplement the early part of an anaesthetic for caesarian section with very low concentrations of an inhalational anaesthetic agent (remembering that halothane relaxes the gravid uterus and may cause a serious haemorrhage). Even so there is often still an appreciable incidence of awareness (1–2%) on the part of the mother during this stage of the procedure. No intravenous analgesic agent is given until the umbilical cord is clamped. Once the baby is delivered the requirements are those for any general anaesthetic for major surgery, the only additional problems being the danger of continued haemorrhage from the uterus (for which oxytocic drugs are given) and the danger of vomiting and regurgitation on recovery.

Chapter 22

Anaesthesia for Eyes, ENT and ECT

OPHTHALMIC SURGERY

The special problems associated with ophthalmic surgery are those related to
1 the site of the operation,
2 the avoidance of rises in intraoccular pressure particularly when the globe is open, and
3 the occulo-cardiac reflex.

Site of operation

In the days before routine endotracheal intubation, this was a major problem, with the anaesthetist trying to keep the patient asleep and the airway patent using bulky apparatus close to the field of operation. Most ophthalmic operations were consequently done under local anaesthesia. With endotracheal intubation this is no longer a problem but, with the patient covered with drapes, access to ensure the security of the airway and for monitoring purposes is limited.

Intraoccular pressure

Any factors that raise intraccular pressure must be avoided. If intraoccular pressure rises when the globe is open during, for example, cataract surgery, vitreous may be extruded and the sight of the eye subsequently damaged or lost. Factors raising intraoccular pressure include any sort of straining, coughing, and vomiting, retching, respiratory obstruction, and even the presence of an endotracheal tube in the pharynx and larynx.

An elevated Pco_2 also raises intraoccular pressure. Post-operative vomiting after the globe of the eye has been closed is not so serious but it is still undesirable and many would choose to give an anti-emetic routinely. Active steps can be taken before, during and after the operation to reduce intraoccular pressure. These include hyperventilation, deepening the anaesthetic and the administration of acetozolamide to inhibit secretion of the aqueous humor.

The occulo-cardiac reflex

This is seen particularly during squint surgery in children. When the surgeon pulls on the eyeball a profound bradycardia may be produced by reflex vagal stimulation and this can cause a cardiac arrest. It is prevented and treated by the administration of atropine.

OTORHINOLARYNGOLOGICAL SURGERY

Like ophthalmic surgery, one of the problems of ear, nose and throat (ENT) surgery is the need of surgeon and anaesthetist to have access to the same area. It is compounded in this instance by them both actually working in the airway. Again the problem is largely solved by the use of an endotracheal tube, this time passed through the nose or fixed in place in the mouth by a special 'gag' so as not to get in the surgeon's way. Additional problems arise from the danger of respiratory obstruction and the presence of blood in the airway post-operatively, particularly if the patient has not fully recovered control of his pharyngeal reflexes. Local anaesthetic spray to the pharynx and larynx prior to intubation should be avoided in order to maintain the integrity of the laryngeal reflexes post-operatively. Many ENT operations are of short duration and surface analgesia may persist into the post-operative period. The patient should be nursed in the 'tonsillar position' after operation so that any blood in the mouth drains out through the nasopharynx rather than entering the respiratory tract. Any anaesthetic technique should allow for rapid return of consciousness. Post-operative vomiting, coughing or straining of any sort will put up venous pressure and increase the possibility of post-operative haemorrhage.

ELECTROCONVULSIVE THERAPY

This type of psychiatric treatment is now normally carried out under a brief general anaesthetic and muscle relaxation using only an induction agent, and the short acting depolarizing muscle relaxant suxamethonium. This makes the treatment more bearable for the patient and decreases the likelihood of fractures due to the accompanying muscle contractions. The problems are those of administering anaesthesia usually at a site distant from the main operating theatre — with all its supporting services, monitoring, resuscitation equipment and recovery room facilities — on a population who are often elderly with an appreciable incidence of intercurrent cardiac and respiratory disease. The muscular contractions that occur with the convulsion, although alleviated in their severity by the muscle relaxant, increase oxygen consumption and, if the patient has not been well ventilated with oxygen prior to the treatment, this may make him hypoxic. In addition the muscle contraction associated with the convulsion may make him difficult or impossible to ventilate.

Chapter 23

Dental Anaesthesia

Dental practitioners were amongst the pioneers of general anaesthesia and thus have inherited their right to practise anaesthesia. Surprising as it may seem, it is not illegal for a dentist to induce general anaesthesia and then extract teeth. The dangers of this practice are so obvious that it has been abandoned by all but the most reactionary and bold. Over the last decade there has been a noticeable fall in the number of patients requiring general anaesthesia for dental extractions — a consequence perhaps of dental education and fluoridization of drinking water. Even so, over one million dental anaesthetics are given annually in Britain.

INPATIENT TREATMENT

Patients for major dental procedures, or patients with systemic illness are treated as inpatients. Dental anaesthesia under these circumstances follows the usual practice for head and neck surgery with conventional premedication and nasotracheal intubation. The procedure is carried out with the subject supine, and blood and tooth debris is removed by an assistant armed with a sucker.

OUTPATIENT TREATMENT

The vast majority of dental anaesthetics are given in private dental practitioners' surgeries, or local authority dental clinics. Although the recent trend has been increasingly to use the supine position, there are many dentists who still prefer to extract teeth from a sitting patient — it is claimed that leaving tooth fragments and blood in the airway is less likely with the sitting posture. The main problems, therefore, are consequent upon anaesthesia in the sitting subject who is also an out-patient. The difficulties recently have been compounded by dentists offering lengthy conservation treatment under general anaesthesia.

TECHNICAL CONSIDERATIONS

Most dental surgery anaesthesia is achieved without endotracheal intubation using a nasal mask. With the mouth open the anaesthetic gases need to be supplied to the nasal mask under positive pressure to avoid too much dilution with air breathed through the mouth. Most traditional dental anaesthetic machines provide an intermittent gas flow which is supplied by triggering a demand valve with the negative pressure of an inspiratory effort.

Nitrous oxide/air anaesthesia was always associated with severe degrees of hypoxia. Even nitrous oxide/oxygen anaesthesia, due to the low potency of nitrous oxide, can result in hypoxia. With the current acceptance of at least 30% oxygen at all times, most dental anaesthetists either add halothane to the inspired mixture or use i.v. agents — especially methohexitone. If halothane is used, a 'draw-over' vapourizer is placed so that all inspiratory gases pass through it. The vapourizer, unlike a Fluotec, must have a low resistance to gas flow.

ANAESTHESIA

A rubber mouth prop is often inserted between the teeth before induction so as to avoid the use of the potentially damaging mouth gag.

Mouth breathing is reduced by carefully layering a cotton gauge or cellulose pack at the back of the mouth. This pack also protects the airway from tooth fragments, blood and saliva.

Anaesthesia needs to be fairly deep as tooth extraction is painful enough to 'break through' light levels of anaesthesia. With intravenous drugs, the patient is likely to be either apnoeic or at least have depressed respiration, which discourages absorption of nitrous oxide. If halothane is used to provide adequate anaesthesia, the patient will often sleep for a considerable time after completion of the extractions. Yet rapid re-awakening is desirable for all outpatients, especially when there remains the possibility of aspiration of blood.

Maintenance of the airway is often difficult. The dentist, when working on the lower teeth, usually pushes the mandible backwards and obstructs the airway. The anaesthetist and dentist strive for a dynamic equilibrium which is just short of airway obstruction. During this battle the anaesthetist must observe the vital signs as best he may. He can palpate the pre-auricular pulse and directly observe respiration though it is often impossible to measure the BP.

COMPLICATIONS

1 Hypoxia can result from too low an inspired Po_2, airway obstruction or drug-induced respiratory depression; the former is unlikely with modern dental anaesthetic machines or Entonox.
2 Mouth breathing lightens the level of anaesthesia significantly. Although nitrous oxide is a low potency anaesthetic it is a very effective analgesic — 25% nitrous oxide is more potent than 10 mg morphine i.v.
3 Airway obstruction is a constant problem. With i.v. induction using methohexitone, the larynx is very sensitive to irritants such as blood and saliva, and laryngeal spasm can result.
4 Aspiration of foreign material which is often infected can result in lung abscess. If a tooth or tooth fragments are aspirated, bronchoscopy should be performed as soon as possible.
5 In lightly anaesthetized patients the 'pain' of extraction causes catecholamine release and arrhythmias often result.
6 Fainting in the sitting position is liable to cause gross cerebral ischaemia and brain damage. Fainting is probably vasovagal in origin, though other causes of hypotension would produce a similar clinical result. Fainting can be prevented by atropine.
7 Excitement is not a feature of modern dental anaesthesia as inhalational inductions are rarely used.

SPECIAL DANGERS AND DIFFICULTIES

Patients anaesthetized in private dental surgeries often suffer from inadequate pre-operative assessment of medical problems. A dentist will often ask the patient's GP to inform him whether the patient is fit for a general anaesthetic; yet the GP himself is no expert. Pre-operative ECG and chest X-ray will not be easily available, nor will a routine haemoglobin be measured in most patients.

The lack of facilities can be critical if things go wrong. Most older anaesthetic machines are not fitted for IPPV. Most dental surgeries do not yet have an electrical defibrillator, nor an ECG machine. The drugs an anaesthetist might need in a crisis will not normally be kept in a private dental surgery as the dentist will have to buy these drugs himself. The anaesthetist must go with all he might require including endotracheal tubes, laryngscope, etc.

Patients with an apical abscess present the inexperienced anaesthetist with major potential difficulties. The trismus, so often a feature, may not be relieved by a muscle relaxant if it is caused by direct stimulation of the muscle tissue by local toxins. Usually the posterior oral region will be swollen with brawny oedema, and the laryngeal inlet is often difficult to see during laryngoscopy due to oedema. When the offending tooth has been extracted, the airway may become soiled with pus.

CONSERVATIONAL DENTISTRY

Many different techniques using a variety of drugs have been tried. Each technique has its proponents who are naturally enthusiastic.

Intravenous diazepam given incrementally until the patient's eyes become droopy is followed by a weak mixture of nitrous oxide. Intermittent intravenous methohexitone is another fairly common method. Some anaesthetists are prepared to maintain anaesthesia with halothane.

After any of these methods the patient is likely to experience drowsiness for many hours.

Chapter 24

Intractable Pain Therapy

For the last 25 years there has been a slow but progressively increasing awareness of the need to treat intractable pain in specialized centres. This has developed with the emergence of practical techniques and the introduction of drugs capable of modifying not only pain itself but also secondary manifestation of it.

Traditionally pain is thought of as a symptom of a disease process, and ideally its control is achieved by controlling or eradicating the disease causing it. The treatment of the underlying disease is rarely undertaken in a pain clinic, and when a treatable disease is suspected the patient is referred to the relevant specialist. Thus, patients receiving treatment in a pain clinic usually have been referred after a diagnosis has been undertaken. A closed pain clinic is restricted to referrals within the hospital, whereas an open clinic accepts patients directly from general practitioners and hospices for the terminally sick. Patients referred from outside the hospital represent a greater challenge as the diagnosis of the underlying disease is often less certain.

The treatment of pain as a symptom has gradually moved from being solely the responsibility of the GP to involve a variety of specialists including neurosurgeons, psychologists, rheumatologists and anaesthetists; services are also provided by orthopaedic, dental and general surgeons. Most pain clinics are organized and run by anaesthetists many of whom have developed operative skills previously restricted to neurosurgeons, such as cordotomy, hypophysectomy and trigeminal ganglionectomy.

DRUG THERAPY

Non-steroidal anti-inflammatory analgesics

Drugs of this type include preparations of aspirin, and other antiprostaglandin compounds including piroxicam and indomethacin. Most of the drugs in this group are particularly good for musculoskeletal and joint pain. They are also very valuable when used with opiates in metastatic malignant disease to reduce local inflammation. They are liable to cause gastrointestinal complications including nausea, mucosal ulceration and haemorrhage. Indomethacin and certain other similar agents can cause headache and a sensation of lightheadedness which can prove to be dangerous when given to machine operatives.

Minor opioids

There is an increasing number of synthetic opioid analgesics which have a more pronounced analgesic activity than the anti-inflammatory drugs. The group includes codeine derivatives, dextropropoxyphene, pentazocine, buprenorphine and nalbuphine. The latter three drugs are partial agonists which also have antagonist activity, and should be combined with opioid agonists with care. Buprenorphine is available as a sublingual tablet. These drugs have less side effects than the opiates causing little respiratory depression, though nausea can be marked, especially in the ambulant subject.

Major opioids

These agents are reserved for severe pain, especially of a visceral type, and pain associated with terminal disease as they induce a useful degree of euphoria. A valuable recent addition is an oral sustained-release morphine preparation which need only be given 12 hourly. Most patients require 50mg b.d. corresponding to 2 mg/hour. For i.m. use heroin has one major advantage over other opiates as it is much more soluble and so the volume required is appreciably less. This is important when heroin is given i.m. to a cachexic individual with terminal disease. Respiratory depression is a problem for short-term use and addiction for prolonged use.

Other drugs

1 Some types of pain of central nervous origin, including post-herpetic neuralgia, can be treated effectively with one of the anticonvulsants such as carbamazepine or sodium valproate. The mechanism of these drugs may be to depress abnormally active central nerve cells which have been affected by the disease process.

2 Systemic steroids greatly help patients with terminal malignant disease, producing both anti-inflammatory effects and euphoria.

3 Tricyclic antidepressants, especially when combined with phenothiazines, have valuable analgesic activity coupled with elevation of mood. Most patients with intractable pain become depressed.

4 Phenothiazines have several useful activities including sedation, anxiolysis and anti-emesis. All relax muscle and control itching.

5 Anti-emetics are usually required for patients receiving large doses of opiates. There is a large selection including phenothiazines, benzodiazepines, metoclopramide and domperidone. Anti-emetics act at different central and peripheral sites. It is often necessary to try several to obtain full relief.

6 Other useful drugs include beta adrenergic antagonists, and dantrolene and baclofen which relieve muscle spasm.

PRACTICAL PROCEDURES

Somatic nerve blocks

1 Pain caused by peripheral nerve entrapment due to localized oedema or fibrosis can be reduced by infiltration with a solution containing a local anaesthetic and a corticosteroid. With somatic nerve entrapment due to a prolapsed intervertebral disc, infiltration of the epidural space is often very effective.

2 When a peripheral nerve is frozen using a percutaneous cryoprobe (freezing probe), loss of all nerve function occurs until the nerve axon regenerates. Pain sensation frequently does not return. The sites for cryoanalgesia include intercostal nerves, abdominal nerves, certain sensory nerves supplying the limbs, such as the lateral cutaneous nerve of thigh, and the pudendal nerves.

3 Peripheral nerve function can be abolished permanently using a local infiltration of either 5% aqueous phenol or 50% alcohol.

4 In metastatic malignant disease involving the pelvis, glycerinated 5% phenol can be injected into the subarachnoid space so that only the posterior (sensory) nerve roots are destroyed; this requires careful positioning of the patient and often results in sphincter disturbances which may be permanent. This type of treatment should be reserved for the terminally sick.

5 Application of heat using a radio frequency generator and percutaneous probe, in which there is thermistor for monitoring the temperature, can be used to produce a localized nerve lesion. Painful vertebral facet joints can be denervated with this procedure. This technique can also be used for percutaneous cordotomy of the lateral spinothalamic tracts, and the fractional destruction of the trigeminal ganglion in patients with trigeminal neuralgia.

6 Surgical section of the nerve proximal to the pain-producing lesion can be a very effective method of obtaining pain relief but is often technically difficult.

Sympathetcomy

Certain types of diffuse pain can be carried in autonomic nerves. Blockade or destruction of part of the stellate ganglion can relieve pain in the head, neck and upper limb. The coeliac plexus can be approached as it surrounds the coeliac axis in the upper abdomen, and this is used to control upper abdominal pain such as with chronic pancreatitis or carcinoma. The lumbar sympathetic chain, situated on the anterolateral aspects of L2, 3 and 4 vertebrae in the retroperitoneal space, can be destroyed to control lower limb pain especially of ischaemic origin.

Nerve stimulation

Pain relief with counter irritation has been used for centuries. The modern equivalent is the transcutaneous electrical nerve stimulator (TENS) which is a device transmitting electric pulses of short duration through the skin via carbon/rubber electrodes. The placing of the electrodes is largely empirical and pain may only be abolished during stimulation, although many patients experience continuing analgesia for a time afterwards. It is possible to implant electrodes close to the dorsal columns of the spinal cord.

Miscellaneous

Acupunture is undoubtedly effective in some types of pain, possibly through the release of endorphins, the naturally occurring opioids.

Hypnotherapy is only effective in a small percentage of patients and requires special experience and time on the part of the therapist. Autohypnosis can be learned by some patients. Physiotherapy provides a variety of treatments including heat, traction and exercises which are valuable for patients with joint or muscle pain.

PSYCHOLOGICAL PAIN

Much of what has been suggested so far in this chapter refers to pain of organic origin. Yet many patients experience pain or abnormal sensations which seem to originate in the central nervous system without any obvious organic cause. This can sometimes be demonstrated by using epidural local anaesthetics diagnostically to see if a peripheral pain persists when the area is analgesic. Thalamic pain is a severe and diffuse type of pain that originates in the basal nuclei and is most often encountered in patients who have suffered a cerebrovascular accident.

Apart from thalamic pain, central pain is often assumed to have a psychological aetiology. It is, however, no less real or less distressing for being psychological, but clearly treatment with analgesics and nerve block is quite inappropriate. Clinical psychologists are trained to provide help in this type of problem and they use various analytical and behavioural methods which are beyond the scope of the present discussion.

It should be appreciated that the patient with organic pain can also benefit from a psychological assessment, and neurotic patients can have organic disease.

Index